A Disease of Society

A Disease of Society

Cultural and Institutional Responses to AIDS

Edited by

DOROTHY NELKIN
DAVID P. WILLIS
SCOTT V. PARRIS

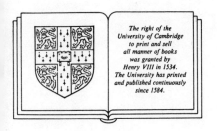

The right of the
University of Cambridge
to print and sell
all manner of books
was granted by
Henry VIII in 1534.
The University has printed
and published continuously
since 1584.

CAMBRIDGE UNIVERSITY PRESS

Cambridge

New York   Port Chester   Melbourne   Sydney

Published by the Press Syndicate of the University of Cambridge
The Pitt Building, Trumpington Street, Cambridge CB2 1RP
40 West 20th Street, New York, NY 10011, USA
10 Stamford Road, Oakleigh, Melbourne 3166, Australia

© Cambridge University Press 1991

First published 1991
Reprinted 1991

Printed in the United States of America

Library of Congress Cataloging-in-Publication Data

A Disease of society: cultural and institutional responses to AIDS/
edited by Dorothy Nelkin, David P. Willis, Scott V. Parris.
p. cm.
ISBN 0-521-40411-8 (hard) – ISBN 0-521-40743-5 (pbk.)
1. AIDS (Disease) – Social aspects.   I. Nelkin, Dorothy.
II. Willis, David P.   III. Parris, Scott V., 1951–
RC607.A26D56   1991
362.1'969792–dc20   90–15071
                                                                        CIP

British Library Cataloguing in Publication Data

A disease of society: cultural and institutional responses to AIDS.
1. Man. AIDS. Social Aspects
I. Nelkin, Dorothy.   II. Willis, David P.   III. Parris, Scott V.
362.1042

ISBN 0-521-40411-8 hardback
ISBN 0-521-40743-5 paperback

Quotation from Paul Monette, *Love Alone,* St. Martin's Press,
New York, 1988. By permission of St. Martin's Press.

Contents

Acknowledgments

We began work on this volume in 1988 with the fervor of ency-
clopedists. The very nature of the acquired immunodeficiency syndrome
(AIDS) epidemic invites critical inquiry into—and from—so many
branches of human learning that no less an effort seemed justified.
Many individuals thoughtfully challenged us to expand the scope of
our effort: Barry Adam, Dan Beauchamp, Jeanne Brooks-Gunn, John
D'Emilio, Don DesJarlais, Richard Dunne, Zillah Eisenstein, Miriam
Fine, Alexander Forger, Ronald Frankenberg, Samuel Friedman and his
colleagues at Narcotic and Drug Research, Inc., Frank Furstenberg, Jr.,
John Gagnon, Bert Hansen, Gregory Herek, Evelyn Fox Keller, John
Martin, Cliff Morrison, Gerald Oppenheimer, Robert Padgug, Monroe
Price, Lillian Rubin, Nancy Scheper-Hughes, Claire Sterk, Steven Tip-
ton, Paula Treichler, and Etienne van de Walle.

Difficult choices had to be made; the fruits of this initial selection
were published as supplements to *The Milbank Quarterly* in 1990. Further changes—additions, revisions, and updates—led to the current
volume.

Two persons who have remained characteristically modest and anonymous, but without whom this volume could not have been completed,
merit our special thanks: Clive E. Driver and Norman L. Wiltsie.

Introduction: A Disease of Society
Cultural and Institutional Responses to AIDS

DOROTHY NELKIN, DAVID P. WILLIS,
and SCOTT V. PARRIS

A IDS IS NO "ORDINARY" EPIDEMIC. MORE THAN A devastating disease, it is freighted with social and cultural meaning. More than a passing tragedy, it will have long-term, broad-ranging effects on personal relationships, social institutions, and cultural configurations. AIDS is clearly affecting mortality and morbidity—though in some communities more than others. It is also costly in terms of the resources—both people and money—required for research and medical care. But the effects of the epidemic extend far beyond medical and economic costs to shape the very ways we organize our individual and collective lives.

Social historians in recent years have pursued their studies of epidemics beyond the charting of pathogenesis and mortality to explore how diseases both reflect and affect specific aspects of culture. In writing about nineteenth-century cholera, for example, historian Asa Briggs (1961) called it "a disease of society in the most profound sense. Whenever cholera threatened European countries it quickened social apprehensions. Wherever it appeared, it tested the efficiency and resilience of local administrative structures. It exposed relentlessly political, social, and moral shortcomings. It prompted rumors, suspicions, and, at times, violent social conflicts." Similarly, historian Gordon Craig (1988) observed: "It was no accident that preoccupation with the dis-

1

ease [cholera] affected literature and supplied both the pulpit and the language of politics with new analogies and symbols."

The literature describing the impact of AIDS is burgeoning. But most studies have focused on the medical and social epidemiology of the disease: how, for example, the virus entered the population and how it spread to different groups. Those analyses that deal with institutional responses suggest how norms and values have influenced various aspects of AIDS epidemiology and the efforts to control and to treat the disease; that is, the ways in which social values have shaped specific efforts to deal with the disease and its consequences. These contributions—for example, on public health agencies (Bayer 1989), public schools (Kirp 1989), the U.S. Public Health Service (Panem 1988)— have been central to our understanding of the past and present forms of the epidemic.

But AIDS will also *reshape* many aspects of society, its institutions, its norms and values, its interpersonal relationships, and its cultural representations (Bateson and Goldsby 1988). Just as the human immunodeficiency virus mutates, so too do the forms and institutions of society. Current clinical, epidemiologic, demographic, and social data about AIDS suggest that the future will be unlike both the present and the past.

How can we grasp the complexity of a society's response to disease? We need, surely, to avoid the tendency among many contemporary scholars and analysts to approach social problems by relying on public opinion polls or surveys, which may "confuse . . . cultural history with market research" (Lasch 1988). Rather, we must explore the accommodative process between disease and social life in its multiple dimensions, and the language and images that mediate their interaction. As the effects of the epidemic—and the numbers of persons infected— widen over the next five, ten, or twenty years, there will be many changes in our social institutions. Some will be adaptive and temporary, likely to change again; others will be more permanent, structural, and likely to persist.

Our intention in this book is to explore the impact of AIDS on American culture and institutions from the perspective of the humanities and social sciences. The notion of culture, as we embrace the term, is an elusive concept. In past decades culture has been conceptualized as a complex but relatively coherent and enduring "web" of beliefs, meanings, and values. Recently, however, scholars have emphasized the truly volatile nature of cultural constructs. Political scientists write of "fragile values," referring to the very tentative and recent cultural acceptance of the rights of homosexuals, women, and various ethnic groups (McKlosky and Brill 1983). Sociologists studying the social construction of knowledge reject the concept of "enduring values," arguing that situations, interests, and organizational pressures influence cultural definitions (Berger and Luckmann 1966). Contemporary anthropologists write of the "predicament of culture," thinking of culture "not as organically unified or traditionally continuous, but rather as negotiated present process" (Clifford 1988). They argue that changes in technology and communication affecting patterns of social mobility and migration have substantively reshaped culturally accepted ways of thinking and acting.

AIDS demonstrates how much we as a "culture" struggle and negotiate about appropriate processes to deal with social change, especially in its radical forms. The contributions in this volume suggest that the institutions we have created to provide social and health services, make laws, enforce regulations, and represent ourselves in the arts and media are less monolithic and more malleable than we generally suppose. In confronting AIDS and its sequelae, these institutions are compelled by external and internal pressures to re-examine their objectives, operations, or methods, and to adapt in order to remain functional, effective, or meaningful. Clearly, no change stemming from this process is permanent. Rather, AIDS induces us to keep appraising the complex and fluid array of benefits and risks that may result from pursuing particular courses of action.

Social Perceptions of Risk

AIDS appears at a time when risks to health are a priority on the public agenda. The effects of toxic substances, chemical wastes, pesticides, food additives, and radiation are a persistent source of fear. We are preoccupied with health—with biological fitness, diet, and exercise regimes. We are bombarded with "data" about risks and benefits, and confronted with seemingly impossible choices. Even the egg—once a symbol of aesthetic design and nutritional perfection—is now the "Trojan Egg." "There are no risk-free lunches. Or breakfasts. Or dinners," say the health authorities (Hanson and Bennett 1989). But then, we are even losing our unquestioning trust in authority—government bodies, medical organizations, scientific experts—to protect our health. Metaphors of contamination and pollution, of death and dying pervaded cultural discourse in the 1980s and persist today.

The public fear of AIDS reflects more general risk perceptions. Psychologists suggest that the characteristics of risk will influence their acceptability; that people underestimate familiar risks and overestimate those that are unfamiliar, involuntary, invisible, and potentially catastrophic (Fischoff, Slovic, and Lichtenstein 1979). Anthropologists emphasize the political, cultural, and social factors that influence risk perception (Douglas 1985). Attitudes toward risk are often subjective, embodied in a complex system of beliefs, values, and ideals. Thus, different social groups will emphasize certain risks and minimize others, or perceive similar risks in quite different terms (Nelkin and Brown 1984). Most important for the analysis in this volume, perceptions of risk are closely connected to moral principles (see the chapters in this volume by Ronald Bayer, Thomas H. Murray, and Thomas B. Stoddard and Walter Rieman). A judgment about risk can be a social comment, reflecting points of tension and moral conflicts in a given society.

In the case of AIDS, social and moral issues have compounded technical uncertainties. There is little consensus about the extent of danger, and still less about the nature of evidence or the court in which the facts are to be adjudicated. Is fear of AIDS irrational or justified by the actual risk? Are experts to be trusted or are they suspect? And, in fact, who are the experts? Nor, in the context of changing values, is there consensus about the appropriate responses to this disease. Despite strong scientific agreement that AIDS is not transmitted through casual contact, controversial proposals—enforced quarantine, mandatory screening, closing of gay bars, constraints on marriage and childbearing, and exclusion of infected persons from work, restaurants, and schools—have been fueled by prejudice and fear. AIDS, to some, symbolizes the problems posed by the dramatic challenges to traditional values that began in the late 1960s, developed during the 1970s, and still polarize the public.

When people see their "way of life" at risk, they characteristically become less tolerant of social differences. In their quest for order and control, they construct distinctions between normal and perverse, legal and criminal, innocent and culpable, healthy and diseased. Labeling AIDS as a disease of certain groups becomes a way to focus blame, to isolate the sources of contamination and contagion, and to deny the vulnerability and responsibility of the wider population.

Social Tensions and the Quest for Order

This quest for order reflects certain social and political tensions that are inherent in American culture. Our very nationhood and its defining Constitution are premised upon the ebb and flow of conflicts; they are never resolved, only checked and balanced. Many of these tensions have shaped, and will continue to shape, the response to AIDS in an array of social institutions — schools, prisons, the military, hospitals, the law, the church. Institutions address dissension in ways that reflect their ideology and professional ethos. But ideology and ethos themselves are not "organically unified or traditionally continuous." AIDS has been not only a catalyst for change in a continuing process of institutional and professional adaptation, but also a source of visible strain. Debates over many institutional and professional tensions — once largely confined to boardrooms, governing councils, journals, and courts — are now more often conducted in open and ad hoc forums. They are diversely, and often graphically, expressed in cultural representations through art and entertainment, music, and the media.

Certain values in American society have always been contested. We prize individual autonomy *and* social order, for example. Both are important to our personal and collective lives. Yet, increments to one value often compromise the other. Similarly, we prize both free choice *and* equity, but these too exist as dynamic constructs rarely, if ever, poised in equilibrium. And we value cultural diversity while imposing conforming norms. The tensions in American values are reflected in a set of questions that recur as we seek to deal with AIDS:

- *What is society's commitment to individual autonomy when communitarian values and objectives are at risk?* AIDS exacerbates the latent tensions between individual rights and social goals, as the need to protect the public health confronts the norms of privacy and confidentiality in personal life. Americans voice support of civil liberties, but often reject their concrete application. Even within the realm of private relations, such contradictions lead to interpersonal tensions: an infected person's "right to confidentiality" is pitted against the partner's "right to know"; the infected woman's right to "reproductive choice" is poised against the right to be "well born." Social policies may constrain an individual's reproductive choices in ways recalling the eugenic policies of an earlier age. Such tensions are at the heart of Ronald Bayer's essay.

• *What are the limits of tolerance about nonconformity to mainstream values?* Only in recent times have we as a society come — very tentatively — to accept a variety of sexual orientations and life styles. AIDS has put new strains on public tolerance, reflecting old struggles between puritanism and hedonism. Our society today exploits — even markets — certain aspects of sexual behavior, while it also condemns those who practice them. Thus the association of AIDS with sexual behavior has subjected some individuals to stereotype and stigma while deflecting attention from the vulnerability of others. Richard Goldstein, in his chapter on cultural representation of AIDS, characterizes this as a tension between the "implicated" and the "immune." Writing on discrimination, Thomas B. Stoddard and Walter Rieman address the legal implications of the tensions over social and sexual conformity.

• *What are the appropriate roles and responsibilities of government in managing disease?* The federal government was extraordinarily slow in recognizing the seriousness of AIDS, so that state and local government first assumed primary responsibility. Even then, traditional strains over respective responsibilities in a federal system, and public ambivalence about appropriate interventions, obstructed concerted action. Debates over government involvement have continued in discussions of both therapeutic measures and public health policies. Observe, in the chapter by Harold Edgar and David J. Rothman, the changing views of risk as the Food and Drug Administration (FDA), a normally conservative organization, has begun to remove procedural obstacles to the availability of innovative therapies. Note the debates over the government role in dispensing free needles, promoting sex education in the schools, and closing bathhouses. Far less contentious, and surprising to many observers, has been an emerging congressional consensus about the resources needed to treat those with AIDS. However, the belated appropriation of federal emergency relief funds to hospitals is unlikely to avert further crisis in those cities and states hardest hit, especially in the public hospital systems where the demands of AIDS compete with the compelling needs of other diseases.

- *What are the roles and responsibilities of the "family"?* AIDS places family relationships—between parents and children, between married and unmarried partners—under intense strain. The disease has mirrored the confusion caused by changing definitions of the family and shifting assumptions about its role. The United States Bureau of the Census has documented the extraordinary variety of nontraditional patterns of household formation, including those of single individuals, pair bondings, and cohabitating but otherwise unrelated adults. AIDS, as Carol Levine's chapter shows, gives poignancy to these impersonal findings. It underscores the changing role of the family as a reproductive unit and the difficulty of developing socially sensitive approaches to adolescent sexual behavior, reproductive choice, and contraceptive use. Tensions arise between the experimentation of teenagers convinced of their invulnerability to physical and sexual "accidents," disease, and even death, and the efforts of adults to temper their behavior.

- *What are the roles and responsibilities of professionals?* The constant struggle among equally honored yet competing values in the society has complicated professional roles and responsibilities. Charles L. Bosk and Joel E. Frader show how AIDS aggravates conflicts inherent in the professions. The physician, for example, traditionally honors a professional duty to several, often conflicting, parties—to science, to the primacy of the patient, to the society at large, and, importantly, though not always explicitly, to his or her self-protection. AIDS has challenged the relative priorities among these values; self-protection, for example, has become an unprecedented concern in the course of clinical practice. The disease has also challenged the hierarchical relationships in hospitals. In the past, specialization in medicine has increased professional dominance. Nurses, paraprofessionals, and volunteer groups inevitably have subordinate social status, reflected in social tensions and low morale (Freidson 1970). Their critical participation in the care of AIDS patients may be a source of change. Now, as Renée C. Fox, Linda H. Aiken, and Carla M. Messikomer observe, the nursing profession has opportunities to reestablish the importance of its caring mission.

Institutional Responses to AIDS

The chapters in this book illuminate in the American context the responses to these and other tensions dramatized by AIDS. And they suggest possible directions for change as we confront AIDS in the future. Social responses over the past decade have ranged from denial to heroic action, from apathy to creativity, from withdrawal to activism, and from prejudice to promotion of communities of shared identity. By understanding the present social context and current strategies of adaptation and accommodation, we aim in this book to shed light on a continuing social process.

Richard Goldstein opens the analysis by examining the epidemic's extraordinary impact on our cultural vision. Some works in the fine arts reflect the perspectives of the "implicated," that is, people with AIDS or human immunodeficiency virus (HIV) infection; others, especially those in popular forms of entertainment, represent the views of the "immune." AIDS in art is an emblem of the involved "insider" or the stigmatized "other." The two themes embody enduring tensions between different approaches to social life. Yet, some television and commercial films have begun to portray AIDS from the "implicated" perspective; more Americans, Goldstein suggests, are coming to experience the epidemic closer to home.

We then explore the changes AIDS has evoked in three systems of socialization and control—the family, prisons, and regulatory agencies. These three institutions' experiences with AIDS—and other social upheavals—testify to their capacity for change when confronted with profound threats to their normative character or hegemony. Jurisdictions across the country have reinterpreted what constitutes a family when those individuals responsible for each other's health and welfare, through affirmed affectional commitment and adoption as well as kinship and marriage, press for recognition of the functional similarity of these bonds. As the incidence of HIV disease has risen sharply in correctional facilities, some jail and prison officials have been forced to deal with the reality of drug use and same-sex intercourse in their midst—and to take (thus far, extremely limited) steps to improve health care and health education in those facilities. The FDA has now approved a "parallel track" system for expanded use of experimental drugs for AIDS, a procedure that loosens the agency's direct control over monitoring drugs' safety and effectiveness.

As more people live in nontraditional arrangements, Carol Levine observes, the gap between their needs and official designations of the "family" has widened. AIDS has exacerbated tensions over the family, affecting legal definitions, medical decision making, and questions of child custody and housing rights. Existing families must adapt to the exigencies of AIDS: changing laws and customs may condition how new families form. HIV disease threatens the intimacy and acceptance ideally characteristic of family ties, yet at the same time reinforces their necessity.

Nancy Neveloff Dubler and Victor W. Sidel report that AIDS heightens long-standing tensions over jurisdictional matters in jails and prisons, including issues of health care. Despite court decrees that the incarcerated have a constitutional right to health care, judicial decisions have often expanded correctional officials' discretionary powers, effectively limiting delivery of many AIDS services. Inmates and parties representing them have thus brought suit against correctional authorities over basic problems of inadequate medical treatment, overcrowding, and drug use in urban and rural facilities. How we care for incarcerated people today, Dubler and Sidel state, will directly affect future use of community services for AIDS and other conditions.

AIDS is also evoking new policies and practices in drug regulation and usage. Harold Edgar and David Rothman argue that the rigorous procedures developed by the FDA prior to the 1980s to minimize risks to human subjects is changing in order to maximize innovation. The FDA is hastening access to investigational drugs and easing drug importation for personal use. In effect, decisions about benefits and risks are being transferred to patients and their physicians — a policy with far broader implications for the entire medical care system.

Our next section explores how AIDS bears on tensions over the role of health care professionals and service providers. The three chapters offer complementary portraits of those dealing with AIDS on the front lines of medical and political battles, and reveal in depth the conflicts nurses, physicians, and voluntary associations and their members face over professional, organizational, and personal objectives. The "culture of caring" that nurses bring to bear on the epidemic, Renée Fox, Linda Aiken, and Carla Messikomer note, can make a palpable difference in patients' lives. Indeed, the nursing profession has been prominent in organizing systems of care for people with AIDS. Many nurses testify to the redeeming significance they find in their work, but caring for AIDS

patients is also stressful. It remains to be seen whether nursing's visible
contribution to creating and managing forms of care will endure.

AIDS, along with other institutional factors, is also remolding the
"shop-floor" culture of house officers and students in urban medical
centers. Charles Bosk and Joel Frader relate how, prior to the epidemic,
medical workers felt powerless and exploited within the system, yet
proud in their clinical coups and generally physically invulnerable. Ar-
riving at a time of heightened economic competition in medical settings, the HIV epidemic subjects house officers to still more demanding
schedules, increasing their sense of powerlessness and limiting their
possibilities of professional achievement. Fears of contagion, mean-
while, are eroding assumptions of invulnerability in the medical
workplace.

Suzanne Ouellette Kobasa treats the voluntary associations formed to
respond to AIDS as an example of Tocqueville's classic model of American associations, defining and providing services beyond the government's compass. Particular organizations have had considerable — possibly
unique — success in influencing government policies. Yet voluntary associations face daunting challenges of tending to newly affected groups,
devising new tactics to pressure official bodies, and avoiding bureau-
cratization or fragmentation.

Our final section focuses on the epidemic's effects on current debates
about American rights and reciprocities. All three chapters, albeit in
different ways, question how society as a whole is reckoning with individuals' and groups' desire to exercise their rights and privileges in the
face of AIDS. How do we balance a collective interest in seeing a child
born well with a woman's right to reproductive freedom when she carries HIV? How are we to preserve a sense of national solidarity when we
restrict certain groups from giving blood to the community at large,
even though tests let us detect HIV's presence in specific donations?
How are we to extend Fourteenth Amendment rights to counter the
contemporary diversity and complexity of bias, including discrimination against people with HIV infection? Each chapter, in short, illumi-
nates how AIDS is contributing to reframing the American social
contract.

Ronald Bayer shows how the specter of pediatric AIDS challenges assumptions about women's reproductive freedom. Many health officials
hold that HIV-infected women should not become pregnant. But this
conflicts with the views of genetic counselors, feminists, and medical

ethicists who want no more than nondirective counseling concerning reproductive choice. AIDS is forcing American society to confront increasing tensions over the limits of liberal individualism in the sphere of reproduction.

In his chapter on "the poisoned gift," Thomas H. Murray addresses the effect of AIDS on the system of blood donation. Patients and physicians now understand that blood carries risks and should not be used unless necessary. Blood banks, initiated as a communal service, have developed new priorities. Some individuals are saving or pooling their own blood for future reuse, while particular groups are targeting donations. The "gift of blood" has become a powerful symbol of community for many, of exclusion for others.

Finally, Thomas Stoddard and Walter Rieman remind us that AIDS is the first public health crisis to arise after the civil rights movement. As we seek ways to limit HIV transmission, people who are sick or at risk are often targets of discrimination. Yet, government officials—judges, legislators, and administrators—have to a remarkable degree exercised restraint, reflecting their increasingly sophisticated understanding of the problem of discrimination and the principles of civil rights. Experience with AIDS may further refine ideas about individual rights, especially the Constitutional right of "equal protection under the law."

AIDS is reshaping many other dimensions of social and institutional life beyond those we could directly address in this volume. Most obvious are changes underway in the lives of gay people. A great deal has been studied and written about the diverse culture commonly referred to as the "gay community"—its putative epidemiologic role in AIDS and its extraordinary adaptations to confront the epidemic (Altman 1986; Shilts 1987; Padgug 1989). Indeed, these adaptations—from personal responsibility and collective activism to greater openness about the vast repertoire of human sexual practices—have recast our vision of the possible. Widely accepted limitations on voluntary behavior change have been challenged and often redefined by the community's campaigns for "safer sex." The ongoing efforts of the community for self-determination and self-help—at first a lonely struggle for self-preservation—have defined our local and national paradigms for care. In a sense, the gay community has come to represent the apotheosis of community action and consumer hegemony. Virtually every institution with which we deal has been catalyzed by these responses.

The measures taken by the gay community have been chronicled most effectively by its own members. Less has been written to enhance our understanding of the social dynamics, rituals, and practices among intravenous drug users—and of the tensions within that "community." Here, we are more dependent upon outside observers and analysts (Friedman et al. 1990). Even less attention has been given to women. As recent congressional investigations document, women have been virtually excluded from scientific study. The media, too, have generally ignored the complex dilemmas of women at risk (Treichler 1987). This situation, however, is fluid as activist and articulate members of this "community at risk" find their voice.

AIDS is clearly changing the practices of many institutions as they try to contain the incidence of disease within their domains. It is re-opening to intense scrutiny the way health care is organized, baring competing claims between "mainstream" and "dedicated" (once called "segregated") approaches to services. It is forcing professional associations in health and social fields to devise informed and humane approaches to AIDS research. And it is impelling scientists, pressured by the urgency of illness, to turn attention to AIDS, and sometimes to alter standards for experimental evidence. Many investigators have responded, with benefits accruing not only to AIDS/HIV research, but also to the basic sciences of virology, immunology, microbiology, and molecular biology. Advances in managing infectious disease, oncology, neurology, pulmonary medicine, and disorders of the immune system are notably attributed to what has been learned from AIDS (Office of Technology Assessment 1990).

AIDS is also challenging the media as they confront an alert, educated, and committed readership in the gay community that sees public communication as politically essential to its goals. It is prompting political parties to forge workable planks on AIDS education, treatment, and approaches to cure. And, finally, it may change, perhaps in drastic ways, the policies of such diverse bodies as insurance companies, regulatory agencies, immigration authorities, employers, churches, and especially, public health departments. The traditional functions of public health departments—to protect health, to maintain law and order, and even to promote economic stability—were so closely related in cholera-stricken Paris in 1832 "that all three influenced the framing of every piece of public health legislation. In other words, health legislation had objectives that extended beyond health per se. Both the government and the governed viewed health legislation in terms of its broader effects . . . " (Delaporte 1987). Such interconnections are apparent today as people and organizations adapt in America's AIDS-stricken cities.

The chapters in this volume deal with only some of these issues, but they suggest that institutions address challenges in ways that flow from their cultural traditions and social imperatives. Each chapter demonstrates an aspect of the very process Clifford (1988) identifies as "negotiating the present." Equally important, however, is what these chapters imply for negotiating the future. The epidemiology and demography of AIDS will change — often unpredictably and harshly so. But the cultural and institutional responses to this disease of society will also change. With the insight, compassion, and vigilance suggested by our authors, these responses may also be enlightening and liberating.

References

Altman, D. 1986. *AIDS in the Mind of America*. Garden City, New York: Anchor/Doubleday.

Bateson, M.C., and R. Goldsby. 1988. *Thinking AIDS*. Reading, Mass: Addison-Wesley.

Bayer, R. 1989. *Private Acts, Social Consequences*. New York: Free Press.

Berger, P.L., and T. Luckmann. 1966. *The Social Construction of Reality*. New York: Doubleday.

Briggs, A. 1961. Cholera and Society in the Nineteenth Century. *Past and Present: A Journal of Historical Studies* 19 (April):76–96.

Clifford, J. 1988. *The Predicament of Culture: Twentieth-century Ethnography, Literature, and Art*. Cambridge: Harvard University Press.

Craig, G.A. 1988. Politics of a Plague. *New York Review of Books* 35 (11):9–13.

Delaporte, F. 1987. *Disease and Civilization*. Cambridge: MIT Press.

Douglas, M. 1985. *Risk Acceptability According to the Social Sciences*. New York: Russell Sage.

Fischoff, B., P. Slovic, S. Lichtenstein. 1979. Which Risks Are Acceptable. *Environment* 21 (May):17–38.

Freidson, E. 1970. *Professional Dominance: The Social Structure of Medical Care*. New York: Atherton Press.

Friedman, S.R., D.C. DesJarlais, C.E. Sterk et al. 1990. AIDS and the Social Relations of Intravenous Drug Users. *Milbank Quarterly* 68 (Supplement 1): 85–109.

Hanson, A.A., and W.I. Bennett. 1989. Trojan Eggs. *New York Times Magazine* (July 30):25–26.

Kirp, D.L. 1989. *Learning by Heart*. New Brunswick: Rutgers University Press.

Lasch, C. 1988. Reagan's Victims. *New York Review of Books* 35 (12):7–8.

McKlosky, H., and A. Brill. 1983. *Dimensions of Tolerance: What Americans Believe about Civil Liberties*. New York: Russell Sage.

Nelkin, D., and M.S. Brown. 1984. *Workers at Risk*. Chicago: University of Chicago Press.

Office of Technology Assessment, U.S. Congress. 1990. How Has Federal Research on AIDS/HIV Disease Contributed to Other Fields? Staff paper no. 5. Washington.

Padgug, R. 1989. Gay Villain, Gay Hero: Homosexuality and the Social Construction of AIDS. In *Passion and Power: Sexuality in History*, ed. K. Peiss, C. Simmons, and R. Padgug, 293–313. Philadelphia: Temple University Press.

Panem, S. 1988. *The AIDS Bureaucracy*. Cambridge: Harvard University Press.

Shilts, R. 1987. *And the Band Played On: Politics, People and the AIDS Epidemic*. New York: St. Martin's Press.

Treichler, P. 1987. AIDS, Homophobia, and Biomedical Discourse: An Epidemic of Signification. *October* 43 (Winter):31–69.

Part I.

Cultural Images

The Implicated and the Immune

Responses to AIDS in the Arts and Popular Culture

RICHARD GOLDSTEIN

W HEN AIDS FIRST PENETRATED AMERICAN consciousness back in 1981, few cultural critics were prepared to predict that this epidemic would have a broad and deep impact on the arts. But ten years later, it is possible to argue that virtually every form of art or entertainment in America has been touched by AIDS. Every month, it seems, more is added to the oeuvre of art, dance, music, and fiction inspired by the current crisis. Not even tuberculosis, that most "aesthetic" of epidemics, produced a comparable outpouring in so short a time.

Though epidemics have played a major role in shaping American society, artistic production in response to devastating periodic outbreaks of yellow fever, cholera, and influenza (not to mention consumption) has been all but indifferent. There is no great American novel about the "Spanish Lady" that killed millions in the years following World War I; no revered poem or play commemorating the evacuation of a major American city due to rampaging disease; no major motion picture about the polio epidemic that swept the nation in the 1950s. Nothing in American literature is comparable to the preoccupation with pestilence that had inspired great works of European realism by writers as diverse as Defoe, Ibsen, Mann, and Camus. Taken as a whole, American culture's response to epidemics—from Edgar Allan Poe's "Masque of the Red Death" to Sinclair Lewis's *Arrowsmith* and

17

Hollywood melodramas like *Jezebel*—has been romantic and didactic. We have wanted to see these outbreaks as anomalous and otherworldly — something occasioned, if not caused, by self-indulgence and other signs of moral laxity.

How different from this stilted silence is our response to AIDS. The current epidemic is the subject of dozens of novels, essays, plays, and poems: family sagas like Alice Hoffman's (1988) *At Risk* and Robert Ferro's (1989) *Second Son*; elegies for lost loved ones like Paul Monette's (1988a,b) companion volumes, *Love Alone* and *Borrowed Time*; blistering critiques like Larry Kramer's (1985) *The Normal Heart*; pastoral evocations of the risk-free past like Andrew Holleran's *Ground Zero*; and intimate accounts of the uncertain present like *The Darker Proof*, a collection of stories by Adam Mars-Jones and Edmund White (1988). In addition to these works, there has been a profusion of polemics, from Susan Sontag's (1989) erudite deconstruction of *AIDS and Its Metaphors* to the more radical *AIDS: Cultural Analysis/Cultural Practices*, an anthology of activist/academic writing edited by Douglas Crimp (1987). Larry Kramer set the standard for the fierce neo-Ibsenism of many plays about AIDS, but there have also been intimate dramas such as William Hoffman's (1985) *As Is*, bold attempts to reconcile sexuality with survival such as Robert Chesley's *Jerker*, and, more recently, even musicals. *Falsettoland* (1990), the sequel to William Finn's *March of the Falsettos*, has an AIDS motif buttressing its claim to moral seriousness. The commercial success of plays about AIDS suggests that the audience for dramatic works about this epidemic is broad. AIDS has been felt across America as a dark presence if not an actual disease, and art has followed the trail of the unfathomable. Alan Bowne's play *Beirut*, in which New York is imagined as a city divided between the infected and the well, is one example of the many works in which AIDS becomes a metaphor for the quality of ordinary life in the 1980s.

AIDS: Catalyst for Cultural Response

The cultural response to AIDS was initially literary, but in the last few years there have been newly composed requiems, symphonies, dances, and performances, as well as painting, photography, videography, and installation art. (Indeed, the intrusion of AIDS into the iconography of

contemporary art is startling enough to have inspired the recent controversy between the National Endowment for the Arts and an exhibition space in lower Manhattan that mounted a provocative show of
works about the epidemic. It might also be argued that AIDS has sen-
sitized the art world to the significance of sexuality as a subject,
thereby fueling the recent congressional ban on federal funding of "ob-
scene art.") Almost as extraordinary as their candor is the range of formal strategies and thematic concerns these works embody. Some artists
have taken utterly traditional aesthetic stances, in an attempt to vali-
date an emotional bond between gay men that is almost as reviled as
their desire, while others have opted for postmodern text-and-image,
in an effort to intervene in how the epidemic is perceived and to generate political activism. This outpouring of work in so many genres and
styles has placed AIDS at the forefront of the arts: a stunning departure from our traditional obliviousness to epidemics and their significance. So extensive is the current response that the 1989 International
Conference on AIDS in Montreal found it necessary to include a series
of presentations on SIDART [this acronym combines the French equivalent for AIDS with art].

One reason for this explosion of interest is the population in which
AIDS was first identified. It is often supposed that homosexuals are, by
nature, artistic, and, in fact, AIDS has taken an appalling toll among
gay men in the creative disciplines. But the arts have also served as an
arena in which homosexuals can address—and redress—the inequities
of their social status. When AIDS struck, this complex involvement
with creativity became a powerful weapon for a community under medical and political siege. The arts enabled gay men to bear witness to
their situation, express feelings of grief that society often distorts, and
create a model for communal solidarity, personal devotion, and sexual
caution that would be necessary to combat a sexually transmitted disease with no known cure.

No comparable process of self-expression exists among the other
groups hit hardest by AIDS—IV drug users, their children, and their
mostly black or Hispanic partners—in part because of the paralyzing
impact of poverty and stigma among these groups, in part because
there is no "community," perceived as such, to bind drug users together. In their isolation and secrecy, these people with AIDS are far
less visible than the middle-class white homosexuals whose plight has
been so amply documented. Pregones, a bilingual troupe that performs

highly evocative dramas in New York, is one of a few theater groups
that represents the distinct experience of Hispanics with AIDS, their
lovers, and their families. Recently, activist videographers have attempted to circulate their work in facilities that serve people of color,
providing a more empathetic, and more directly experiential, view of
AIDS in "the other America." But much of the work directed to minority audiences is funded by hospitals and social service agencies. Its
thrust is largely pedagogic, its concerns are often incomplete (the crucial subject of bisexuality in these communities is rarely broached), and
its reach is limited. AIDS is increasingly a disease of impoverished people of color. Yet, if one were to describe this epidemic from works of
art alone, one would have to conclude that only white women and gay
men have been people with AIDS.

The Implicated and the Immune

Popular culture has found itself drawn to depictions of the causes and
consequences of HIV infection. The epidemic's image in movies, popular music, comedy, and television is very different—though no more
accurate or inclusive—than its representation in the arts. These two images reflect quite distinct cultural responses. The first, located in the
arts, is focused on people with AIDS, portraying them with a nuanced
complexity intended to compensate for social stigma by "implicating"
its audience in the epidemic. The other carries the perspective of the
mass media; it presumes to be objective or, in terms more suited to
this discussion, "immune." This mass cultural response is largely concerned with the society surrounding people with AIDS: the spouse,
children, family, friends, and colleagues of the infected. A host of distinctions follows from this shift in point of view.

The arts attempt to tell the "story" of AIDS from the inside out.
The protagonist is presumed to be innocent and is seen, if not in isolation, than in the solitude of a heroic relationship. Stigma and survival
are regarded with equal seriousness, and the artist struggles to give the
person with AIDS a fully human complexity. He (sometimes she) is a
kind of everyperson, struck at random and often rendered more, not
less, typical by the disease. One senses in much art about AIDS a
familiarity with its subject, as if the artist were immersed in dealing
with the epidemic—as so many are. Many of the best works about this

disease have been produced by people at various stages of HIV infection. Perhaps they are struggling with disease, or have lost a lover, nursed a dear friend, or attended a dozen funerals at a young age, and feel themselves to be, in every sense, set apart by the experience. They are implicated. Their art signifies a collective trauma—mass death in the midst of life.

But AIDS in America—more than even other sexually transmitted diseases—has seemed to "select" its victims from among previously defined groups: at first, homosexuals and IV-drug users; more recently, women of color and their children. Though, in fact, no one who is sexually active can be presumed immune to AIDS, the progress of this epidemic (and the technology that enables us to assemble a perceptual pattern of its spread) has given AIDS in the West the quality of a selective blitz. That, in turn, has made it possible for mass culture to assume the perspective of a "witness" to AIDS who also stands outside it. This second cultural response—unbounded by direct experience of the epidemic—reflects the fears and fantasies of those who regard the world of AIDS as emblematic of the "other." If the arts have positioned themselves with the implicated, the mass media represent the immune.

This point of view makes the image of AIDS in a TV movie vastly different from its representation in painting, choreography, serious fiction, and noncommercial cinema. In television, where demography is destiny, the person with AIDS is rarely an innocent everyman. That category is reserved for infants and young hemophiliacs. Adult males are usually represented as transgressors whose behavior places others in jeopardy; infected women are usually exempt from blame, but rendered nearly as helpless as their children. In these prime-time masques, it is not the person with AIDS who is victimized but those threatened or affected by the disease. Family and community occupy center stage, and the issue is not survival but cohesion: how to deal with a breach in the safety net.

This disjunction between art and entertainment corresponds to the tension between empathy and anxiety that pervades the nation's political response to AIDS. The locus of the epidemic in America has made it possible (so far) to think of this as a disease of subcultures, pitting ancient emblems of stigma and taboo against modern concepts of pluralism and the prerogatives of identity. The AIDS crisis, coming at a time of crisis for American liberalism, seems to signify the clash between contemporary and traditional values. The ambivalence unleashed by this "epidemic of signification," to borrow Paula Treichler's (1987) term, makes it necessary to have not just one cultural response to AIDS, but two of them: one representing the implicated, the other the immune.

AIDS in Film: Representations of Immunity

"AIDS has all the elements for a good movie—drama, passion, tragedy," the film critic Vito Russo, an AIDS activist and a person with AIDS, recently told a reporter. Yet, until recently, only independent films, such as Bill Sherwood's bittersweet gay comedy, *Parting Glances*, dealt more than glancingly with the disease. That film—in its wry, unflinching familiarity with the subject and its determination to place the epidemic in the context of ordinary life—shares the "inside-out" stance of the fine arts. It has taken a decade for that point of view to appear in a Hollywood film—the modestly budgeted and selectively distributed *Longtime Companion* (1990) by Craig Lucas, recently released to movie theaters and scheduled to be shown on public television. The occasional critical jab at Lucas's candor about homosexuality notwithstanding, several major films about AIDS are in development. But this does not change the fact that Hollywood has turned a cold shoulder to people with AIDS. The best-known AIDS drama, *The Normal Heart*, has been optioned by several major stars (including Barbra Streisand), according to its author, Larry Kramer; but the play has yet to be made into a film. In his powerful essay, "Reports from the Holocaust," Kramer (1989) compares Hollywood's obliviousness to AIDS with its failure to make films about the Nazi Holocaust until years after it occurred. Just as Jewish studio heads then conspired in silence, today, gay executives reason: better *Batman* than the boy next door dying of a sexually transmitted disease.

That does not mean, however, that the impact of AIDS has gone unnoticed by Hollywood. A film like *Fatal Attraction*, with its scenario of the adulterous husband who unwittingly brings a voracious killer concubine into his family, evokes the anxieties this epidemic has generated without requiring its audience to confront the lives of homosexuals and drug addicts. Indeed, the entire aura of the sex comedy has changed since AIDS. Now, the swingers envy the stable, and even the unrepentant take precautions, as in the appearance of a glow-in-the-dark condom in *Skin Deep*, a recent Blake Edwards comedy.

But it is horror films—the genre with the sharpest refraction of collective angst—that have responded most vividly to the AIDS aura. Punishment for illicit sex (along with retribution for technological hubris) has always preoccupied American horror films. Indeed, these are the contemporary equivalents of lurid breviaries with images of syphilitics before the judgment of Christ. Those who commit the sin of fornication (or that of Faust) must bear the cost: In the classic observation of horror films, "They tampered with God's will." AIDS has revived a traditional symbol of such concerns: the alien organism that invades the body and transforms it into something terrible to behold. This metaphor for disease, and for ancient images of mortification of the flesh, is updated in *Alien*. Here, an extraterrestrial monster enters the body of an astronaut by literally inseminating him through the mouth—a deft allusion to sodomy—and then bursts forth from his belly, a pathology that clearly relates to the violation of gender roles.

An even more resonant image is provided by *The Fly*, a remake of the 1950s horror classic, in which a mad inventor creates a machine that can transport matter, only to see his own protoplasm contaminated by that of a fly which has entered the machine. Both the original film and its remake offer a critique of scientific hubris, a common horror theme since *Frankenstein*. But the 1980s version also contains a heavy dose of sexual paranoia. A "liberated" woman—often the object of punishment in horror films—has fallen in love with the inventor, but his flylike incarnation shatters her self-confidence: "Be afraid—be very afraid!" she screams. The arrogant inventor has not only become an insect; in the process, he has lost his hair, teeth, digits, even his penis. This is a distinct allusion to the specter of AIDS, a disease often portrayed as reducing handsome young men to monsters with running sores that ooze from their swollen features. To complete the identification with HIV, the inventor's condition is passed on to his son in a sequel, *The Fly 2*. Contaminated genes transform the child, too, into a monstrosity.

One of the ways American culture comes to terms with an unanticipated event like AIDS is to invest it with a scenario that resembles the plot of a horror film. This is the structure of most contemporary journals of the Plague Year, from Robin Cook's (1986, 1987, 1988, 1989) medical fiction to Randy Shilts's (1987) reportage. *And the Band Played On*, Shilts's journalistic history of the epidemic's early years, bears a formal resemblance to a thriller like *Jaws*. Both works feature a lurking leviathan that assaults the unaware at play, while heroic doctors, cast in the mold of Ibsen, do battle with a malignantly indifferent society. Of course, the traditional victim in a horror film is a vulnerable young woman, and the traditional resolution involves destruction of the monster by a virile man. Thus, the fantasy of seduction-by-salvation overcomes our dread of the unknown. But AIDS offers no such denouement. Its shape and scale can only be hinted at in the imprecise terms of epidemiology. Its victims can hardly be characterized, by a society fraught with ambivalence about homosexuality and drug addiction, as innocent young things. And its heroes are anonymous caregivers and activists, engaged in the often thankless task of keeping a vengeful society — along with a monster — at bay.

AIDS in Popular Music and Comedy: Stand-up Hate

Popular forms like rock music and stand-up comedy, which have often served to clarify the terms of social conflict, offer only an oblique image of AIDS. Rock music, whose candor, subjectivity, and youthful audience might have made it the ideal medium for education and opposition to orthodoxy, has dealt with the epidemic primarily in surreptitious (and remarkably crude) asides. The willingness of Madonna to refer to AIDS and condoms in her 1990 *Blonde Ambition* tour is groundbreaking in rock. Rap music, too, has recently incorporated the safe-sex message into its elaborate codes (a condom in this lexicon is a "jimmy-hat"). More typically, though, rock stars rarely refer to the epidemic in their songs; when they do, it is usually in veiled allusions like the one Prince employs when he sings of a friend who died of "a big disease with a little name." Lou Reed's angry eulogy for friends he will no longer see in the Halloween parade is one of the few attempts in rock to acknowledge the reality of AIDS. Indeed, the epidemic threatens the hedonism of rock music in general, heightening resentment against those deemed responsible.

Heavy-metal moralists like Axl Rose of the group Guns 'n' Roses have captured the field of commentary on AIDS in rock music. In a popular lyric, Rose develops homophobic and xenophobic themes. According to the lyrics, "faggots" and immigrants think they are free to act as provocateurs or transmit a "fucking disease" ("One in a Million"[1]

---

[1]Permission to quote the lyrics from "One in a Million" was denied.

1988). At the opposite end of the pop spectrum, the lyrics of "Whatcha Lookin' At" (1990) by the rap group Audio 2 exhort no less violent a response: men who dare to cruise other men will get bashed. What is most shocking about these little ditties is that they appeared in 1988 and 1990. Such sentiments were supposed to have been overcome long ago, after years of awareness about AIDS.

Similar anti-gay invectives have come to permeate the AIDS prevention messages of even the most sophisticated rap groups, reflecting a sexual conservatism that often accompanies black nationalism in America. The politically astute group Public Enemy, for example, offers a decidedly unsympathetic portrayal of gay life in "Meet the G that Killed Me" (1990). The deliberate ambiguity in the song title, referring either to "gay" or "germ," reinforces an ancient conflation of homosexuality and contamination; the rap, in fact, invokes the specter of homosexuality as an unnatural act. When the lyrics provoked angry complaints from gay groups, Public Enemy asserted that homosexuality is a product of Western civilization and did not exist in Africa before Europeans arrived. The image of deviance and disease as an alien import is a mirror of the notion some conservatives put forth that AIDS is a product of bizarre sex practices in Africa.

Radio "shock jocks" have added people with AIDS to their litany of FM abuse. Rush Limbaugh devotes a segment of his show to the epidemic, scored to songs like "I'll Never Love That Way Again." A sub-rosa repertoire of jokes continues to express the onus of a terrified and self-righteous populace. In some circles, "gay" has come to stand for "got AIDS yet?," and the disease itself — renamed "WOG" for "wrath of god" — is referred to as an illness that can "turn an animal into a vegetable." When rumors flew that Richard Pryor was dying of AIDS, the comedian denied them, insisting the slander had been spread by his former wife, who "doesn't want me to get laid anymore." The comedian Eddie Murphy draws material for his act from the reinvigorated stereotype of homosexuals as vectors of disease. In one routine, Murphy refuses to date women who kiss their gay male friends, lest that contact give him AIDS. Murphy's homophobic japes are more than matched by Sam Kinison, who asserts that gay men spread lies about the need to use condoms in order to repress the heterosexual libido, and blames the spread of HIV from animals to humans on the propensity among homosexuals for "screwing monkeys."

These scabrous routines, and others, have drawn huge appreciative audiences, proving that, though the official culture condemns such sentiments, they persist because they correspond to enduring anxieties. As is often the case in comedy, insecurities about sexual identity are at the core of this humor-of-rage. Gay men are the "other," yet they may infect others, suggesting that the distinction between homo- and heterosexual desire may be less firm than we acknowledge. In response, gay men have developed jokes of their own to describe their precarious position. "Hi mom, I've got bad news and good," went one joke of the early 1980s. "The bad news is, I'm gay. The good news is, I'm dying." In another perceptive jab at the fluidity of stigma, some gay men asked each other: "What's the hardest thing about having AIDS? Trying to convince your mother that you're Haitian."

Rock music and stand-up comedy, which once stood for sexual and social revolution, now reflect fear of contagion and rage at the "other." AIDS is not the only reason for this shift, but the epidemic has clearly played a part in aligning these forms with conservative social values. The audience for rock and stand-up-comedy — as well as horror films — is young and mostly male. For this cohort, bombarded by contradictory information about abstinence and safe sex, AIDS must seem especially unfathomable: a disease of junkies and queers that anyone can contract; a scourge that transforms its victims into the "other," depriving them not only of vitality but also of identity. The paradoxical image of AIDS is compounded by society's ambivalence toward its victims: they are labeled sinners, yet are perceived as fully human, even heroic. Rock and comedy, not to mention Hollywood films, have been unwilling to risk alienating their audience by dealing with such a paradoxical tableau.

AIDS on Television: A Matrix of "Immunity"

With other popular forms unwilling to decipher AIDS, the task has been left to that most didactic American medium, television. Initially, this "story" was considered too contentious and too complicated for the prime-time market place. With the death of Rock Hudson in 1985, however, TV news executives abruptly discovered the "human-interest" aspect of AIDS. They realized that uncertainties about who might be at risk could draw a huge audience. The spectacle of young men dying in their prime, of a disease that often wasted their bodies, offered an opportunity for television to represent the gay community without seeming to condone its practices. Sympathy for the afflicted could be enlisted as a device to shift onus away from both sexual deviancy and social bias. Television used AIDS to construct the perspective of the immune, allowing the American people to confront gay men at their least threatening and most affecting.

As it became apparent that the audience for AIDS programming was huge, made-for-television movies about the epidemic proliferated and many dramatic series wove motifs about AIDS into their story lines. The show *Midnight Caller* has run two episodes about a woman suffering from AIDS, who happened to be the hero's former lover. The first installment was devoted to dealing with a bisexual man who had knowingly infected her; gay groups objected strenuously to the premise, persuading the show's producers to alter the ending, so that the hero contemplates, but rejects, vigilantism. The second episode focused on the "victim," using her experiences as a device to get at the plight of people with AIDS. Despite its controversial — and quite banal — aspects, this show epitomizes many of the conventions TV drama has adapted in dealing with AIDS: the victim is a white, middle-class woman, the perpetrator a transgressive male, and the mode of transmission heterosexual. This is hardly the typical cast and scenario of AIDS in America today: most sexual transmission has occurred between men; most women have been infected from IV drug use or from sex with an addicted male (not a bisexual); and the overwhelming proportion of heterosexual transmission cases has occurred among women of color.

The image of the epidemic on prime-time TV is skewed by political and demographic considerations. Showing blacks or Hispanics as people with AIDS might fuel stereotypes about these groups and exacerbate racial tensions; in any event, it would certainly raise concerns among civil rights groups. The result, tragically, may have deprived black and Hispanic women — especially in urban areas — of crucial information about the actual extent of their risk. TV news shows do not misrepresent the epidemiology of AIDS, but neither have they emphasized the facts about who is at risk; and TV movies about AIDS — which carry all the paradigmatic power of popular fiction — invariably focus on whites. Since homosexuality is easily as contentious as race, at least where representation is concerned, TV movies about AIDS shy away from gay male protagonists. To focus on drug addiction would make it difficult for the producers of these films to build sympathy for the afflicted: a hallmark of TV movies about any illness. Consequently, the typical protagonist is a young, virtuous, and vulnerable woman: the traditional emblem of innocence. This device has another advantage. It corresponds to the demands of the primary audience for TV movies: women. This demographic base is very different from the mostly male audience for rock music or horror films, and it fosters an image of the epidemic quite distinct from what prevails in those other forms.

Films about the ordeal of families faced by one member's illness are immensely popular in prime time—indeed, terminal illness is an adventure the whole family can enjoy—and, when that illness is AIDS, the presentation is skewed by what programmers perceive to be the perspective and concerns of women. If young men are expected to evince a fear and loathing of homosexuals, the female audience is thought to have a more tolerant attitude. Therefore, people with AIDS (even when they aren't gay) are generally more sympathetically drawn in TV movies than in other popular forms. This characterization is especially true when the protagonist is what one TV movie referred to as *The Littlest Victim* (the original title, *The Most Innocent Victim*, was changed under pressure from gay and AIDS activists). Hemophiliac children are the most common heroes of AIDS movies, and stories about Ryan White and the Ray family (whose home in Florida was firebombed) have drawn large audiences.

Women are not portrayed much differently from "the littlest victims." They, too, have had suffering and stigma inflicted upon them, often by the deceit of men. Offstage stands the prostitute, frequently identified as the source of infection, though, in reality, relatively few cases have been traced to that source. In *Intimate Contact* (a British TV movie shown in this country on the Home Box Office cable network), Claire Bloom plays a prosperous suburban housewife whose life is shattered when her husband is diagnosed with AIDS and confesses his dalliances with prostitutes. This scenario, whatever its relation to reality, transforms AIDS into a crisis for the family, introducing the message of monogamy in stark dramatic terms. (Alone among significant works of fiction about AIDS, Alice Hoffman's [1988] novel, *At Risk*, has a single mother, whose daughter was infected by a transfusion, as its protagonist. By turns touching and horrifying, Hoffman's novel is an antidote to the bathetic conventions of TV movies. But, like the characters in prime-time weepers, everyone in *At Risk* is suburban and white.)

Casting the epidemic in strictly heterosexual terms avoids the wrath of activists, but this convenient dramatic device also avoids confronting the actual contours of AIDS, and creates a false impression that everyone is equally at risk. On the other hand, if the protagonist of an AIDS movie were a gay male, the networks might arouse the wrath of religious fundamentalists — unless the "victim" were cast in an offending light, which would offend gay viewers, not to mention many women. As a result, the commercial networks have produced only one major film about a gay man with AIDS. *An Early Frost* remains a highly instructive paradigm of how popular culture deals with both the problem of deviance and the anguish of premature mortality.

As this made-for-television film opens, the hero lives apart from his family with another man. When AIDS strikes, he returns home — the faux household of a gay couple is revealed to be a fragile shelter that must give way to the enduring arms of mother, father, sister, and grandma. Unfortunately, father is repelled by his son's homosexuality, and most of the action in the film occurs between these men, as the women struggle to effect a reconciliation. To them falls the task of caring for the doomed deviant, and, though sis has some initial reservations about allowing her brother to touch her baby, the victim soon finds himself enveloped in a cushion of love, and even father relents when he realizes what lies ahead. This is not an implausible story, nor is it ungenerously told, with sympathetic portraits of other gay men, including the former lover and an AIDS patient who dies courageously but alone. Still, as this tale unfolds, the protagonist becomes less and less central to the plot. The family, rather than the person with AIDS, is the actual subject of this film.

An Early Frost achieves its ambition, which is to fold the mythography of AIDS into the conflict between father and son. This is a tale in which love overcomes (male) righteousness, and sin is forgiven in the face of death. As the credits roll, the son has been reconciled with his family. He drives off into an uncertain sunset, but the family — through its own capacity to change and grow — coheres. As a model for dealing compassionately with the stigma of AIDS, *An Early Frost* is far from il-liberal. But as a strategy that makes the person in crisis peripheral,

subordinating his needs to broader social concerns, it is hardly empathetic or, for that matter, true to what people with AIDS have struggled to achieve.

Representations of Implication

How different this prime-time scenario is from *Second Son*, a novel by
Robert Ferro (1989), who died of AIDS shortly after it was published.
In this tale, too, AIDS brings the rifts within a family to a head, and
here, too, an obdurate father is forced by his gay son to face himself.
But because this is a novel, free of the populist demands of television,
and because it was written by a gay man who knows his subject well,
the changes wrought by AIDS are far less archetypical. The father never
fully relents, the family cannot transcend the tragedy of the protagonist's illness, and he fails to find solace among them. If the real
subject of *An Early Frost* is the cohesion of the social unit in the face
of an epidemic, the subject of *Second Son* is illness as a catalyst for establishing autonomy. The alternative to family is not, as in *An Early
Frost*, to live and die alone. This gay man finds another man with
AIDS, and as the novel ends, they sit gazing out at the sea, imagining
an endless cruise on a magic ocean liner: the very image of what this
book constructs as a gay male utopia.

Though *Second Son* is hardly a didactic work, one can imagine the
furor if this story of two men with AIDS who find love in each other
ever appeared in prime time. The only "inside-out" representations of
gay men with AIDS have been on public television, where an up-
scale audience is thought to be more receptive to plays like Terrence
McNally's *Andre's Mother* (1990). Similarly, it is only in the more shel-
tered, and segmented, venues of theater, fiction, art, and dance that
gay men have told their side of the story. Art about AIDS has several
important functions within the gay community. It commemorates people whose identity has been stigmatized, compensating for the loss of
social status that often accompanies AIDS by the simple fact of declaring the disease a fit subject for art. It validates bonding between gay
men at a time when such relationships are widely regarded as essential
for survival. It creates an image of the gay community as an agency of
support and nurturance, in contrast to the malign indifference of mass
society. And it seeks to empower people with AIDS, both personally

and collectively, through images that can serve as the basis for political action. Finally, art about AIDS seeks to rescue the struggle for survival from its statistical abstractions by bluntly declaring, as George Whitmore (1989) does in his journalistic account of AIDS in America, *Someone Was Here*.

Even a casual observer of art about AIDS must notice how much weight is placed on love as a counterforce to oppression and death. Much as Larry Kramer's play, *The Normal Heart*, intends to function as a call to arms—and to sexual continence—it ends with an image that would seem to be outside its political agenda: a bedside wedding between two gay men. But this utopian gesture is central to Kramer's social—and sexual—ideology. Throughout his work, devotion is the ideal poised against the twin realities of promiscuity and hostility from the world at large. In William Hoffman's (1988) less strident drama, *As Is*, the mutual caring and acceptance of two ex-lovers (one of whom has AIDS) is all that remains of their formerly baroque sex lives; it makes the present crisis bearable. Even an unrepentantly liberationist playwright like Robert Chesley incorporates bonding into his work about AIDS. In *Jerker* (which nearly cost the license of a California radio station that broadcast segments of the play), a relationship between two men, which exists entirely on the phone, deepens as one of them becomes ill and finally disappears.

Though this emphasis on bonding seems novel, it is a traditional concern of gay male culture, evident in Walt Whitman's concept of "adhesiveness" and E.M. Forster's ([1910]1989) less gender-bound admonition: "Only connect." AIDS has occasioned the recovery of romanticism in many gay representational works—much as tuberculosis fueled operatic masques of purity amid pollution. Once again, death sanctions love and gives it a tragic edge. Once again, a disease is thought to single out the abnormally passionate, creative, and effete. But it is hard to imagine the contemporary gay man as a latter-day Dame aux Camélias. The confrontational stance of today's gay culture gives the bond between people with AIDS in fictional works a more insistent edge. In Paul Monette's (1988b) angry elegy, *Love Alone*, the devotion of two men—one dying and the other infected but well—becomes a cry against death and an affirmation that gay men can love:

I hear how trapped how frantic was my friend / not to go it rings in the wind around me / like a signal sent by a dying star bursting /

here in my dead heart a bloom of black light / calling WE ARE NOT
A MILLION MILES AWAY / SAY WE ARE NOT ALONE...

The same impulse to use traditional imagery of devotion to elevate
and commemorate a gay relationship is evident in "Absence," Bill T.
Jones's dance in honor of his dead lover and collaborator, Arnie Zane.
It opens in a setting that resembles a morgue or hospital. Male dancers,
dressed in flowing white sheets, move with the painful deliberation of
the dying. Then the scene changes: sheets become ballgowns, and the
dancers' racking movements are stately, processional. They move toward the rear of the stage, now bathed in blue light, to Berlioz's
"Nuits d'été." The music, the movement—almost still enough to be a
tableau vivant—and the play of white gowns (on men) against blue
light seem at once campy and utterly funereal. Jones appears, his mus-
cled black body doubled over in laughter. It is the sort of incongruous
image that might well appear in a dream about the death of a lover—
lavish yet aching and somehow concretely gay. Though this dance has
none of the rage of Monette's poetry or Kramer's dramaturgy, like both
these works it uses emblems of high romanticism to eulogize a bond
others might revile. These works, and many others like them, answer
the need to make sense, not just of an epidemic, but of a social status
denied significance.

The de facto and covert nature of gay relationships may have been in
activist Cleve Jones's mind when he came up with an idea for what has
come to be known as the Names Project, a giant quilt the size of several football fields, consisting of commemorative panels prepared by
friends and loved ones of the deceased. Each panel is inscribed with a
name and epitaph or emblematic object—often an image of innocence,
such as a teddy bear, or of transformation, such as glitter and drag—
intended to evoke the person it honors. The allusion is to quilt making:
an American craft traditionally reserved for women, one that connotes
comfort, care, and community. All these concepts are crucial to the
strategy of collective survival, and in that sense, the Names Project
speaks to the living, evoking an image of gay culture in the face of
crisis very different from the assumptions of prime-time artifacts. This
quilt literally contains multitudes, and its sequences of panels are bi-
sected by cloth aisles, so that, when seen in the company of others who
have come to pause, lay flowers, or pray, it resembles an alternative
cemetery.

In the Names Project, as in Bill T. Jones's dance, the methodologies of fine art—in this case, site-specific installation works—are enlisted as a response to social stigma. These panels are modular and mobile, affirming that there will be no official memorial for those who died in this epidemic. Instead, their memory may be carried from city to city, and displayed in shop windows, carried during rallies, or, on special occasions, laid before the White House and the Capitol as a mute reminder of what has been lost. Like the Vietnam Memorial, a sunken slab with names inscribed, this moveable quilt embeds the individual in a collective, commemorating the communal in uncertain times.

The rituals of life and death that have become commonplace in the gay community are rarely recorded by the mass media, which is why the impulse to document them is so strong in art about AIDS. Caregiving, traditionally regarded as a feminine skill, takes on a special meaning for gay men, not just because it defies the traditional rules of gender, but because so many people with AIDS prefer to be nursed by their friends. *A Death in the Family*, a film from New Zealand that has been shown on the Public Broadcasting Service (PBS), borrows documentary techniques to tell a fictionalized story of a gay man dying of AIDS. In *An Early Frost*, the AIDS patient came home to his family, but here, home is where the heart is. The implication is that care provided by peers, in an affirmative environment, is more effective and humane than either institutional nursing or the mercies of a family that harbors conflict toward the person with AIDS. This validation of community is at the core of art that positions itself inside the epidemic—and it is notably missing from much photography about AIDS, raising urgent questions about whether these graphic, sometimes grotesque portraits are to be regarded as artifacts of implication or immunity.

AIDS in Photography: Flashpoints of Ideology

The criticism leveled at photographic representations of AIDS is complicated by the fact that, until recently, many well-known gay photographers shied away from the epidemic in their work. Robert Mapplethorpe, whose death from AIDS is often mentioned in articles critical of his sexual iconography, was reluctant to discuss his own ill-

ness and did not confront it in his oeuvre. Peter Hujar, who took a less
heroic view of gay eroticism, and who graphically represented death
and dying in his work, shied away from AIDS—though Hujar, too,
died of the disease. Activist-photographers like Jane Rossett have produced a more engaged image of the epidemic. Perhaps deliberately,
her work lacks the formal panache of fine-art photography, which remains problematic (at least to many activists) because it often ignores
the social context of AIDS.

Even an empathetic photographer like Rosalind Solomon, who in-
vests her subjects with a determined dignity, shares some of the biases
of mass media. Often, she shows us the person with AIDS embedded
in his or her family, eulogizing the bond between mother and (sick)
child, or (sick) mother and child. Though these images of devotion and
reconciliation are immensely moving, they fail to probe beneath the
familial embrace, or to raise questions about the impact of social structures on the stigmatized individual. Other portraits show people with
AIDS alone, or with their lovers; but even here, the sense of social
struggle is often muted, almost beside the point. For all their artfulness
and verisimilitude, many of Solomon's photographs affirm the domestic paradigm of a TV movie.

Another photographer of people with AIDS, Nicholas Nixon, avoids
the snare of sentimentality by focusing on the individual in extremis.
But his portraits raise another concern, often mentioned in regard to
news photos of people with AIDS as well. The grotesquerie of the disease is evident in Nixon's work, almost as if its real subject were the
process of physical deterioration. Nixon's use of eerie light and stark
framing accentuates this sense of separation from the world. While his
aim is to bypass the interpersonal aspects of AIDS, uncovering the objective processes of life and death (as Nixon has done in other, equally
graphic, portraits of babies, poor people, and the frail elderly), the effect of his stance is to transform the subject into a specimen. The
viewer shares in a voyeuristic spectacle, not unlike the one tabloids rev-
eled in during the early years of the epidemic, when before-and-after
shots of young men in the late stages of AIDS were accompanied by
veiled allusions to the wages of sin. Of course, Nixon has no such
agenda, but some activists maintain that his work reenforces media
stereotypes about people with AIDS. A show of Nixon's photographs—
including portraits of people with AIDS—at the Museum of Modern
Art in 1988 drew protesters demanding, "No more pictures without

context." As critic/editor Douglas Crimp wrote recently, "Part of the context excluded from Nixon's pictures, of course, is everything that kills people with AIDS besides a virus..."

Given the capacity of imagery to shape our perceptions, many artists now presume that representations of AIDS can never be objective. Mere empathy is deemed an insufficient response. The artist is enjoined to compensate for the virulence of stigma by engaging its image in popular culture. The absence of this mediation signals that the artist is not to be counted among the implicated.

The Deconstruction of Immunity

"Witnesses: Against Our Vanishing" is the title of the recent Artist's Space show about AIDS. It includes works by David Wojnarowicz, whose scabrous essay for the show's catalogue, criticizing political and religious leaders, catalyzed the fracas between this exhibition space and the National Endowment for the Arts. Wojnarowicz's art uses found photos as well as drawings and text of his own devising to impose a critical — often homoerotic — perspective on the epidemic. For Wojnarowicz, gay sex is at the core of our terror of AIDS, and the body becomes a prism through which lust and violence are refracted and revealed. Other works in this show — many by women — address similar themes. The casual visitor may conclude that these artworks, in a jumble of media and styles, are merely an attempt to document the emotions of grief and rage, in a variety of postmodern modes. But there is an order to the disorder here, and an underlying sense of mission. The aim is to empower the afflicted by enabling them to deconstruct representations of themselves.

In *Bright Eyes*, a video made for Britain's alternative TV network, Channel 4, Stuart Marshall exhumes the dark tradition of medicalizing homosexuality, juxtaposing images of people with AIDS with nineteenth-century typologies of "moral imbeciles" and "sexual perverts," and placing this legacy against the famous Nazi book burning (which chose, as its initial target, the library of Magnus Hirshfeld, Weimar's most celebrated gay liberationist). Marshall took the title of his video from a caption in a British tabloid ruminating on the sad fate of a once "bright-eyed" gay man with AIDS. The form of *Bright Eyes* — its odd jumbling of dramatization and documentation, its disruptive uses of light and dark tonalities—is meant to disrupt the presumption of objectivity. Fiction and nonfiction are not distinct discourses, Marshall argues. Though medicine and media claim to describe reality, both are heavily weighted with social subjectivity. AIDS is the latest evidence that our conceptions of sexuality and disease are regulated by their representation in science and art.

Departing from the elegiac tone of much gay fiction about the epidemic, works like these are abrasively confrontational. The aim is to produce an alternate AIDS aesthetic, one that undermines the assumptions of mass culture while appropriating the terms of representation. Videographers like Isaac Julien and John Grayson have issued counter-commercials about safe sex, far more affirmative about sexuality (especially homosexuality) than the public service announcements the networks are willing to show. Other videos show people with AIDS in the full bloom of mundanity, living with rather than dying from the disease. The videographer's object is to direct the techniques of documentation toward activist ends, and the target is not just the media's hidden agenda, but the insularity of the art world and its refusal to become engaged. As Douglas Crimp (1987) writes, in his introduction to a special AIDS issue of *October*, the radical art journal: "We don't need a cultural renaissance; we need cultural practices actively participating in the struggle against AIDS. We don't need to transcend the epidemic; we need to end it."

This call to arms has been sounded by Gran Fury, a cadre of commercial artists affiliated with the AIDS Coalition to Unleash Power—better known as ACT UP—who have organized themselves into an art collective that produces symbols and installations to be used in street demonstrations. The ubiquitous "silence = death," framed by a pink triangle from the Nazi concentration camps, functions as an emblem of the AIDS movement. There are also posters, T-shirts, and formal art exhibitions produced by groups and individuals in ACT UP. These "graphic interventions," as Crimp calls them, read very effectively on television and in news photos because their aesthetic is borrowed from advertising and commercial design. Unlike the videos, which are too pedantic and formally evolved to reach a mass audience, art by ACT UP uses the techniques of mass media to deliver a message of dissent.

The impact of this strategy on both popular culture and the fine arts has been significant. Perhaps no artist emblemizes this synthesis more than Keith Haring, who recently died of AIDS. Haring insinuated a message of safe sex and political activism into posters, buttons, and even murals, extending the ACT UP sensibility to inner-city youths, who would ordinarily reject its affiliation with gay liberation. He enlisted his iconography in the struggle against stigma, applying images that connote an energized innocence to slogans associated with AIDS, rendering the epidemic as part of the fabric of urban America. Haring's message, delivered in the ambiguous codes of popular design, is similar to the blunt text of an ACT UP poster, proclaiming, "All people with AIDS are innocent."

There is an ongoing tension between those who think that art—or, as they would call it, "cultural production"—must empower the afflicted, and those who insist on a more subjective—or as they might refer to it, "essential"—response. This conflict is ideological, temperamental, and even demographic. The audience for Edmund White's elegant stories about AIDS might find ACT UP's iconography depersonalized and severe, while activists might find the lush opacity of White's prose indulgent and remote. But both these responses are functional. White's protagonist finds a respite from his overwhelming sense of sterility by having sex with a young Greek hustler (who uses a condom), consoled by the entire history of gay culture in the West. Gary Indiana's (1989) novel, *Horse Crazy*, does not promote a political program but it vividly evokes the current climate of helplessness and horniness, belying those odes to the joy of couplehood that saturate the media (and much gay fiction). Bill T. Jones's dance contains no call to arms, but it addresses the grief and reconciliation that are as much a product of the epidemic as are anger and action. And the Names Project stands against the denial of devotion that is as much a signature of homophobia as is the denial of civil rights. These works are models for mourning and renewal, and they stand alongside the exhortations of ACT UP as elements in a cultural response whose aim is to promote survival, demand attention, and defeat stigma.

This response, coupled with political activism, has been highly effective. Rates of infection have flattened among gay men (at least in large cities). A citizens' movement, unprecedented in medicine, has won significant reforms in the release of new drugs. And the worst excesses of homophobia, which many thought would rise to the fore in the wake of AIDS, have so far been averted. Would the populace have tempered

its initial fear and loathing of people with AIDS without art and action
on the part of activists; and would dramatic changes in behavior have
occurred in the gay community without potent iconography?

In a sense, the power of a coherent cultural response is most evident
in its absence among those who do not perceive themselves to be at
risk. The progress of AIDS among white, middle-class heterosexuals has
been far more subtle than its rapid spread among drug users and gay
men. Indeed, some conservative commentators (e.g., William F. Buckley and Pat Buchanan) have argued that, for drug-free heterosexuals
who do not practice anal intercourse, AIDS does not represent a threat
at all. Safe-sex education has been hampered by religious ideologies,
and the rich potential of popular culture to organize a response to social crisis has been blocked by political constraints. In the face of these
obstacles, movies, music, and media have dealt with AIDS in a highly
inflected manner, offering reassurance in the form of domestic dramas
and warnings in the style of sex-and-splatter films. While these works
are popular, because they deal with collective fears and fantasies, it is
doubtful that they have convinced many people to alter their behavior.
No meaningful attempt is being made to reach teenagers—the group
most likely to think itself invulnerable to sexually transmitted
diseases—though there is increasing evidence that AIDS is spreading
among them in urban areas. Nor has mass culture represented IV drug
users, whose social status makes it impossible for them to represent
themselves. Another group at significant risk—women of color—has
been similarly ignored. Partly as a result of this malign neglect, the
epidemic is growing fastest among these groups. They are, in the language of TV movies, "the most invisible victims": the implicated
among the immune.

Conclusion: Assimilating
the Unfathomable

The question remains: Why has the cultural response to AIDS been so
elaborate? The mere fact that many artists are affected does not account for the profusion and appeal of these works. A fuller explanation
may lie in the distinct anxieties this epidemic aroused. AIDS arrived in
the midst of a moral (and political) panic over sexuality. The assump-

tion that medicine had conquered venereal disease was replaced by an ominous revelation: science could not contain a new and deadly sexually transmitted disease. If anything, technological sophistication added to the anxiety by making AIDS seem unlike any previous pandemic. Here was an illness whose long latency differentiated it from influenza or plague, which could sweep through a population in only weeks. Now, it was possible to ascertain that infection occurred years before the onset of disease. This "diagnosis" created a new class of "patients," forced to live between sickness and health, giving a tangible twist to the old medical term, "worried well." But AIDS anxiety was hardly confined to the infected. Given the vast numbers of Americans who had experimented with sex and drugs during the previous decade—and the cultural backlash against such behaviors—many people outside so-called "risk groups" feared the stigmatization of AIDS.

Both art and entertainment spoke to these anxieties, albeit in very different ways. Mass culture provided a paradigm of social cohesion, while the fine arts offered a model of social struggle. Popular culture gave voice to the fear and rage of the majority, while the arts helped dispel stigma by deconstructing it. Both the fine arts and mass media worked (though certainly not dialectically) to enable Americans to assimilate the unfathomable. Cultural representation, combined with political activism, forged the current consensus on AIDS.

The crisis certainly has not passed. The growing number of women of color (and their children) infected, largely due to heterosexual intercourse with IV drug users, has created a new sense of urgency about bringing treatment and prevention strategies to this population, as well as new demands for restrictions on civil liberties. Already, there are signs of disjunction between mass culture and the fine arts over the representation of AIDS and drugs, just as there has been over AIDS and homosexuality. Activists are still seeking aesthetic strategies that empower the most vulnerable, while entertainers operate from the assumption that both the virus and its carriers must be kept at bay. The struggle to maintain a humane consensus on AIDS continues, and, in the end, that is a political process, not an artistic one.

Signs of polarization remain—in politics as well as culture. The director of a student production of *The Normal Heart* in Missouri recently had his house firebombed; Congress has forbidden federal funding of homoerotic art. No doubt, there will always be a perceptual

gap between the implicated and the immune, but as the epidemic becomes part of ordinary life, one can hope, at least, that the two cultures of AIDS will grow less distinct.

References

Bordowitz, G. 1987. Picture a Coalition. *October* 43:183–96.
Cook, R. 1986. *Mindbend*. New York: New American Library.
———. 1987. *Coma*. New York: New American Library.
———. 1988. *Mortal Fear*. New York: Putnam.
———. 1989. *Harmful Intents*. New York: Putnam.
Crimp, D. 1987. AIDS: Cultural Analysis/Cultural Activism. *October* 43:3–16.
Ferro, R. 1989. *Second Son*. New York: Crown.
Forster, E.M. [1910] 1989. *Howards End*. New York: Vintage Books.
Hoffman, W. 1985. *As Is*. New York: Random House.
Holleran, A. 1988. *Ground Zero*. New York: Morrow.
Indiana, G. 1989. *Horse Crazy*. New York: Grove.
Kramer, L. 1985. *The Normal Heart*. New York: New American Library.
———. 1989. *Reports from the Holocaust*. New York: St. Martins.
Lewis, S. 1962. *Arrowsmith*. New York: Signet Classics.
Mars-Jones, A., and E. White. 1988. *The Darker Proof*. New York: New American Library.
Monette, P. 1988a. *Borrowed Time*. New York: Harcourt Brace Jovanovich.
———. 1988b. *Love Alone*. New York: St. Martins.
Shilts, R. 1987. *And the Band Played on*. New York: St. Martins.
Sontag, S. 1989. *AIDS and Its Metaphors*. New York: Farrar, Straus and Giroux.
Treichler, P.A. 1987. AIDS, Homophobia, and Biomedical Discourse: An Epidemic of Signification. *October* 43:31–70.
Whitmore, G. 1989. *Someone Was Here*. New York: New American Library.

Bibliography

Dance

Absence. Directed by B.T. Jones, Bill T. Jones/Arnie Zane Company, New York, 1989.

Films

Alien. Directed by R. Scott. Twentieth Century Fox, 1979.
Fatal Attraction. Directed by A. Lyne. Paramount Pictures, 1987.
The Fly. Directed by D. Cronenberg. Fly Productions, 1986.
The Fly 2. Directed by C. Walas. Brooks Films, 1989.
Jezebel. Directed by W. Wyler. Warner Brothers, 1938.
Longtime Companion. Directed by N. René. Companion Productions, Inc., 1990.
Parting Glances. Directed by B. Sherwood. Rondo, Yoram Mandell, Arthur Silverman Productions, 1986.
Skin Deep. Directed by B. Edwards. Blake Edwards/Creek Productions, 1989.

Music

"Meet the G That Killed Me." In *Fear of a Black Planet*, by Public Enemy. New York: Def Jam/Columbia, 1990.
"One in a Million." In *Lies*, by Guns 'n' Roses. New York: Geffen, 1988.
"Whatcha Lookin' At?" In *I Don't Care*, by Audio Two. New York: First Priority/Atlantic Recording Corporation, 1990.
New York, by Lou Reed. New York: Sire/Warner Brothers Records, 1989.
Sign of the Times, by Prince. New York: Paisley Park/Warner Brothers Records, 1987.

Photography

Witnesses: Against Our Vanishing (an exhibition). New York, Artists Space, 1989-1990.

Theater

Beirut. By A. Bowne. New York, Westside Arts Theater, 1987.
Falsettoland. By W. Finn. New York, Playwrights Horizons, 1990.
Jerker. By R. Chesley. New York, Sanford Meisner Theater, 1986.
The Lisbon Traviata. By T. McNally. New York, Promenade Theater, 1989.

Video/Television

Andre's Mother. Written by T. McNally, directed by D. Reinisch. Old Fashioned Pictures, Inc., 1990. (Presented on American Playhouse, Public Broadcasting System, 1990.)

Bright Eyes. Directed by S. Marshall. Great Britain, Channel Four.

A Death in the Family. New York, Public Broadcasting Service, 1988.

An Early Frost. New York, NBC, 1985.

Intimate Contact. Directed by W. Hussein. New York, Home Box Office, 1987.

The Littlest Victim. Directed by P. Levin. New York, CBS, 1989.

Midnight Caller (1989–1990 series). New York, NBC.

Part II.

Systems of Socialization and Control

AIDS and Changing Concepts of Family

CAROL LEVINE

A FEW YEARS AGO, AFTER MY DAUGHTER'S marriage, a friend remarked that the wedding had been very unusual. "It was a first marriage," she explained, "and the parents of both the bride and groom were still married to their original partners." Pointing out that my husband and I, unlike most of our friends, had avoided the exquisitely delicate questions of etiquette that complicate the weddings of children of divorced or "blended" families, she asked, "How does it feel to be an anomaly?"

This anecdote may reveal only a glimpse of life among a certain segment of the middle class in New York City in the mid-1980s. There can be no doubt, however, that across the nation American families have changed, are changing, and will continue to change. A statistical snapshot of American families today documents the shifts. Data from the 1980 United States census show a sharp rise from the 1970 figures in the number of single-parent families, nearly all of them headed by women. Almost 20 percent of minors live with one parent, an increase from 12 percent in 1970. The number of people living alone also increased by 64 percent over the previous census. The number of unmarried couples living together almost tripled from 523,000 in 1970 to 1.56 million in 1980, and increased another 63 percent from 1980 to 1988 (U.S. Bureau of the Census 1981, 1988). In 1988, the proportion of households accounted for by married-couple families with children under the age of 18 present in the home had declined by 13 percent since 1970 (U.S. Bureau of the Census 1988). According to the U.S. Department of Labor, by 1987, 64 percent of married mothers with children under the age of 18 were working or seeking work, compared with 30 percent twenty years earlier, and less than 10 percent in 1940 (Levitan, Belous, and Gallo 1988). As Toffler (1980, 211–12) has pointed out, "If we define the nuclear family as a working husband, housekeeping wife, and two children, and ask how many Americans still live in this type of family, the answer is astonishing: 7 percent of the total United States population." That percentage is undoubtedly lower ten years later.

Behind these statistics lie sweeping historical, economic, scientific, and cultural trends. Families are no longer primarily units of production and procreation; they have become instead centers of emotional and social support. Procreation is separated from sexual behavior and is an act of choice rather than necessity. Women, freed from constant childbearing, may choose to enter the labor force. Since they are frequently divorced or never married and are often the sole support of their children, they may have no choice but to enter the labor force.

These statistics are only numerical representations of the extraordinary diversity of family life today. They are based on "household" composition, only one factor used to describe "family." They do not convey the complex and varying arrangements whereby individuals create, dissolve, and recreate supportive and intimate bonds. Tolstoy's (1981 [1877]) famous dichotomous description of families, expressed in the opening lines of *Anna Karenina*—"Happy families are all alike; every unhappy family is unhappy in its own way"—is only half true today. While the second half of the dictum is certainly valid, it is now the case that happy families are not all alike.

In this diverse and shifting milieu a major medical and social crisis encompassing AIDS and HIV disease (hereafter referred to as "AIDS" for simplicity) heightens processes of change already underway and sets in motion new, particularized responses. This chapter is intended to describe some of these changes and to explore their potential impact on current and future families. It is an observational, speculative, nonempirical attempt to call attention to a largely unrecognized aspect of the epidemic rather than to provide a systematic sociological, historical, or anthropological analysis.

While the subject of "family" is difficult to confine within rigid boundaries, this chapter focuses on key intersections where families and societal institutions meet. At these intersections — such as medical decision making, custody decisions, and housing law — definitions of family and rights of family members are straining to accommodate the new situation of AIDS. As Donzelot (1979) pointed out in *The Policing of Families*, the family is not a "point of departure . . . a manifest reality, but . . . a moving resultant, an uncertain form whose intelligibility can only come from studying the system of relations it maintains with the sociopolitical level." In this view families are social as well as biological constructs. In today's world both dimensions of family are being challenged.

Who Counts as Family?

The answer to this apparently simple question is by no means easy. It depends on why the question is being asked and who is giving the answer. "Family" can be used in many ways, from the narrowest interpretation to the most metaphorical, from description to polemic. Consider the recent case of Nancy Klein, a comatose and pregnant Long Island woman. With her parents' agreement, Mrs. Klein's husband, Martin, sought court permission for an abortion, which doctors hoped would improve her chances of recovery. John Short, an antiabortion advocate, sought legal guardianship of Mrs. Klein and her fetus. He claimed, "We are all members of the human family. If we see someone being manipulated into killing a child, we have to step in" (*New York Times* 1989a). In this case, the metaphor of "family" was used to further a political agenda and to override the legal and ethically justifiable decision of a real-life family. The judge ruled in favor of Mr. Klein's request, thus rejecting the claim that strangers who do not approve of medical decisions have a legal right to take decision-making power from traditional family members.

In this chapter I use a definition of "family" that is broad but not unlimited. If everyone counts as family, then family loses its special meaning. If only a few count as family, then our understanding of human relationships is impoverished. What separates family from friends and strangers is not just blood or legal ties but an emotional quality of relationality, continuity, and stability. Individuals are born and marry into families; they also choose to enter relationships that are family-like, even if they are called by other names. The essential characteristics of these relationships are permanence (at least in intention); commitment to mutuality of various forms of economic, social, and emotional support; and a level of intimacy that distinguishes this bond from other, less central attachments. Thus, my working definition is: *Family members are individuals who by birth, adoption, marriage, or declared commitment share deep, personal connections and are mutually entitled to receive and obligated to provide support of various kinds to the extent possible, especially in times of need.* It is perhaps no accident that in the traditional marriage vows, the pledge to remain constant places "in sickness" before "in health"; sickness tests family strength and resiliency as few other crises do. In this context AIDS is the supreme test of family devotion.

This definition both respects traditional notions of family and recognizes nontraditional forms of commitment. Who would be excluded? People in intentionally transitory relationships; individuals who claim status as a family member solely as a convenience to obtain benefits otherwise not available; persons who by abandonment or other actions give up their claims to the benefits of family status. (While a father remains a father, no matter how he treats his child, the recognition that society gives to his status will diminish if he fails to fulfill the minimum obligations of parenthood.) This working definition will undoubtedly be problematic at the boundaries; the central core of deep, long-term, emotional commitment, however, should hold firm.

This definition has some traditional elements. Biological definitions are the most familiar (a word that itself is derived from "family," and connotes shared associations). Dictionary definitions of "family" stress the parent/child relationship. Thus, Webster's dictionary defines family as "the basic unit in society having as its nucleus two or more adults living together and cooperating in the care and rearing of their own or adopted children." Even this definition is being challenged by surrogate parenting, in which a couple commissions a woman to bear the man's child and secures her agreement to give up her maternal rights to the adoptive mother. New reproductive technologies create situations in which a child may have two different "mothers" — one who supplies the genetic material and another who gestates the fetus. It is possible to add a third mother to this complex, if still another woman raises the child.

This working definition further delineates the functional definition offered by the Task Force on AIDS and the Family convened by the Groves Conference on Marriage and the Family:

> Families should be broadly defined to include, besides the traditional biological relationships, those committed relationships between individuals which fulfill the functions of family (Anderson 1988).

Individuals may count as family members people who are unrelated to them in any traditional way; for some purposes self-definition is more important than legal ties. But public policy definitions of family, which determine eligibility for various benefits and privileges, vary considerably from self-definitions. Thus, biologically and statutorily unrelated individuals are usually not eligible for the benefits accorded to spouses and children, regardless of the depth or duration of their emotional or economic attachments.

Legislatures, courts, and governmental agencies differ in defining "family." For example, according to the U.S. Bureau of the Census (1988), "A family or family household requires the presence of at least two persons: the householder and one or more additional family members related to the householder by birth, adoption, or marriage." A householder who lives alone or exclusively with persons who are not related is defined as living in a "nonfamily household." Thus, nontraditional functional and relational coupling of two consenting and committed adults—for example, gay or lesbian couples—are by this definition specifically excluded from the designation of family.

The census bureau's definitions do not directly affect individuals' access to benefits, as do the definitions of some other agencies. There is no single, national legal definition of family; family law is administered by the states, and each state has different definitions. Moreover, definitions adopted by governmental agencies vary, with some being more restrictive than others. For example, the California corrections law limits the people who are entitled to overnight prison visitation with eligible inmates to persons who are related by blood, marriage, or adoption (City of Los Angeles Task Force on Family Diversity 1988, 22). On the other hand, the more broadly construed New York State definition of family in the Domestic Violence Prevention Act includes "persons related by consanguinity or affinity," "persons formerly married to one another regardless of whether they still reside in the same household," "persons who have a child in common regardless of whether such persons are married or have lived together at any time," "unrelated persons who are continually or at regular intervals living in the same household or who have lived in the past continually or at regular intervals," as well as a catch-all category of "other individuals deemed to be a victim of domestic violence as defined by the department in regulation" (New York State, Social Services Law, Section 49(2).

Some people in nontraditional relationships, and some gay and feminist social critics, reject the term "family" because of its historical association with particular arrangements of economic, political, and sexual power that they view as oppressive. Yet the alternatives, such as "bonding groups" and "friendship networks," fail to convey the notion of deep personal connectedness that is suggested by "family." "Community" in some cases — for example, religious communities — does convey this sense, at least for its members. The word is used more commonly, however, to mean a much less central association. While it is important to recognize that family ties can constrain as well as bolster, most people share an understanding of family that suggests a special and enduring, if not necessarily happy, relationship.

As more and more people live in nontraditional arrangements, the distance between their needs and interests and official designations widens. This discrepancy is apparent in many areas, but appears with particular force in AIDS, which, at the same time, heightens the summed impact and lays bare the multiple parts of dysfunctional designations and categories. Those most affected by AIDS and HIV infection — gay men, intravenous drug users and their sexual partners, largely from poor, minority communities — are also those most likely to have nontraditional living or family arrangements. Even if they lived in traditional families before they became ill, the stigma of AIDS and the stress of coping with terminal illness may have created deep intrafamilial rifts. The person with AIDS may thus have to acquire a new family for emotional and economic support. This family may be made up of some traditional family members and friends; increasingly, health care workers and volunteers for social service agencies fulfill the functions of family. In its most extreme and metaphorical version, the hospital becomes the surrogate family. "For many [babies with AIDS], Harlem Hospital is their mother and father. We're all they have," says Margaret Heagarty, M.D., director of pediatrics at the hospital (Breo

1988, 33). Dr. Heagarty, as mater familia, views her wards as claimants to both her relational and functional commitment.

AIDS is a catalyst in efforts to expand the definitions of "family" to reflect the reality of contemporary life. A movement to recognize "family diversity" has emerged in response to the problems experienced by members of nontraditional families, particularly some politically active gay and lesbian couples and elderly unmarried couples, in obtaining benefits such as medical insurance and bereavement leave for their "domestic partners." Starting in Los Angeles, and now spreading to other cities, the organizers call for expanded definitions of family. The City of Los Angeles Task Force on Family Diversity's (1988) final report concluded:

> No legitimate secular policy is furthered by rigid adherence to a definition of family which promotes a stereotypical, if not mythical, norm. Rather, the appropriate function of lawmakers and administrators is to adopt policies and operate programs that dispel myths and acknowledge reality.

In May 1989 the City of San Francisco passed the nation's first law allowing unmarried homosexual and heterosexual couples to register publicly as "domestic partners," thus paving the way for them to obtain health benefits, hospital visitation rights, and bereavement leave. For a fee of $35, domestic partners, defined as "two people who have chosen to share one another's lives in an intimate and committed relationship" can file a "Declaration of Domestic Partnership" (*New York Times* 1989b). This law was revoked by a referendum in July 1989, but will be put to vote again at a later date.

The boundaries and utility for public policy of expanding definitions of family are being tested. AIDS is stretching the boundaries and, by so doing, may change more than definitions. The structures and services of institutions may change in response to the differing arrangements that will be officially counted as "family."

Families in Crisis

AIDS throws families into crisis. Crises in family relationships are often the occasion for bringing private intrafamilial matters to the notice of social institutions that are designed to respond with services and assistance. Because the two groups most seriously affected by AIDS—gay men and intravenous drug users—are generally (and often inaccurately) considered to be isolated from family life, the impact of AIDS on internal family functioning and mental health has not been fully appreciated. Public policy has barely begun to recognize the enormous future needs for mental health and social services that will be needed by persons with AIDS and by their families, however defined. Families are implementers of public policy, sometimes by design, more often by default. A public policy that reduces hospital length of stay for AIDS patients by establishing diagnosis-related groups as the basis for reimbursement assumes that discharged patients will go "home" and that families will provide care. Yet, there are few supports in place to make it possible for families to implement that policy. "Paco," a person with HIV disease, describes this plight:

> To me the problem is that I'm not getting help from anybody else. My parents are doing everything and they can't do it all. And Social Security opens my case and they close it and they open it again (Citizens Commission on AIDS 1989).

This circumstance is not unique to AIDS. For example, there are no explicit employment or tax policies to enable adult children to care for frail, dependent, elderly parents.

Traditional families that have already developed internal ways of coping with crises may be totally unprepared for the stress created by external pressures, such as stigma. Whether the response is rejection or acceptance, as Gary Lloyd (1988), a sociologist of the family, states:

> Families with a member discovered to have HIV infection or diagnosed with AIDS will experience high levels of stress, and disruption in all areas of family life.

Some families, however, react by mobilizing to fight the stigma and are able to transcend their initial fears and prejudices. They may speak publicly about the disease, raise money for research and care, and become advocates for their ill family member and all those affected. One suburban family with seven children was transformed by the experience of caring for a dying gay son; the mother became less concerned with other people's opinions; a sister became politically active; a son who is a physician altered the way he cared for his patients (Tiblier, Walker, and Rolland 1989).

Cultural or religious differences may affect family views. For example, some families have deeply held views against homosexuality or drug use. Nevertheless, in black families a tradition that reveres the mother/child bond may transcend negative attitudes toward these behaviors. Mildred Pearson, a black woman whose son Bruce died of AIDS in 1987, says: "He was a wonderful son. My son was gay. I didn't like that, but he was. He did not leave me any babies or a whole lot of money, but he left me his strength. My son died with dignity" (*New York Times* 1988).

Some Hispanic families, imbued with the concept of *familismo*, accept responsibilities of care for their sick family member, but may be wary of accepting the help of outsiders such as social workers. A counselor in Chicago says, "Latino people are hiding their children and loved ones with AIDS." Part of their reluctance is based on unsatisfactory experiences with non-Spanish-speaking health care workers and, in some cases, a fear of discovery of illegal entry into this country. In addition, many Hispanic families have a deep distrust of doctors and the medical system (*Chicago Tribune* 1987; Nelson Fernandez, personal communication).

Abandonment by families of their sick or disgraced members is a familiar theme in life and literature. Silas, the hired man in Robert Frost's (1971 [1914]) poem "The Death of the Hired Man," goes back to Warren and Mary, his employers, to die. Warren asks his wife: "Silas has better claims on us you think/Than on his brother? . . . /Why didn't he go there? His brother's rich./A somebody—a director in the bank."

While many families have not abandoned a relative with AIDS, irrational fear of transmission added to religious or cultural stigma have led to rejection. Even among Jewish families, often stereotyped as the most protective and supportive of their children, AIDS creates divisions. In 1989, eight years into the HIV epidemic, a New York City congregation held a special, separate Passover seder for its members with AIDS because some of their families were afraid to invite them to the family gathering and risk the wrath of those who wanted no association with AIDS (*Newsday* 1989a).

Because nontraditional families are more commonly socially and psychologically similar to the patient, having been deliberately formed around shared interests, they may be better equipped to respond to external pressures such as stigma, but not to the dependency and level of care occasioned by illness. Most of these family members are young; caring for someone their own age who is dying may be particularly traumatic. Where a number of people are involved, competition for the ill person's reliance and trust may erupt. Susan Sontag's (1986) short story, "The Way We Live Now," depicts such a web of complex interrelationships:

> According to Lewis, he talked more often about those who visited more often, which is natural, said Betsy, I think he's even keeping a tally. And among those who came or checked in by phone every day, the inner circle as it were, those who were getting more points, there was still a further competition, which was what was getting on Betsy's nerves, she confessed to Jan; there's always that vulgar jockeying for position around the bedside of the gravely ill.

In some cases only certain family members are involved in the care and support of the person with AIDS; in others, the roles and functions are shared and rearranged to meet the needs of the moment. In still others, families are in conflict, occasionally or permanently, over issues such as treatment decisions, disposition of property, and funeral arrangements. Within all families, relationships may shift over time, as individuals move in and out of different roles and functions.

Nontraditional Families and Social Institutions: Slouching toward Flexibility

While some families have demonstrated remarkable capacities to adjust to the stress of AIDS, the institutions that serve as their formal social support—the law, welfare systems, health care, insurance, housing—are less flexible. AIDS is only one of many situations revealing the inadequacies of these institutions in responding to the needs of nontraditional families, but because of its high visibility and urgency, it could be a catalyst for change.

American social institutions were constructed with a particular vision of the family that was a dim reflection of the reality of many minority, immigrant, poor, or other families out of the white middle-class mainstream. These institutions are ill prepared to deal with the complex, novel, and highly charged issues presented by AIDS. Their inadequacy is apparent at many points between diagnosis of AIDS and death and even beyond. Courts and other agencies have, however, already had to confront the problem in three areas: (1) decisions about medical treatment; (2) housing; and (3) custody decisions.

Decisions about Medical Treatment

A central focus of the field of biomedical ethics, which began in the 1960s as a response to the biological revolution and the prevailing norm of medical paternalism, has been patient autonomy — the right of competent individuals to make health care decisions for themselves. When the person is unable to make those decisions, either because of illness or legal incompetence, the classic question has been: "Who decides?"

Legal efforts to ensure the rights of individuals to make treatment decisions or to designate a particular person as a proxy have centered on some form of advance directive or "living will." These documents set out the patient's wishes concerning what kinds of treatment are acceptable and under what conditions, and they may designate a person to act as proxy. Thirty-eight states and the District of Columbia now recognize advance directives for treatment decisions (Society for the Right to Die 1987). Eighteen states have legalized the patient's appointment of a durable power of attorney in health care to express the patient's wishes if the patient becomes incompetent (Cohen 1987). While durable powers of attorney are well established in financial matters, their status in health care is less certain, and decisions made by a person designated in this capacity may be challenged.

Although not legally entitled to make treatment decisions, "the family" has generally been considered the appropriate surrogate. In the hierarchy of decision makers, parents are normally considered surrogates for minor children, spouses take on the surrogate role after marriage, and children act as surrogates for widowed, elderly parents. When the family structure does not conform to these patterns, or is not defined by traditional relationships, conflicts among family members, and between family members and physicians or hospitals, may arise. Controversies concerning termination of life supports have been at the center of biomedical ethics discourse.

Bringing a new set of actors—lovers and nontraditional family members—into the equation complicates the decision-making process and sets the stage for conflict. A Minnesota case involving two lesbians has become a symbol for advocates of the rights of women, gay people, and the disabled. Sharon Kowalski, a former high-school physical-education teacher, became paralyzed and suffered brain damage after an automobile accident in November 1983. After the accident the woman with whom she had lived, Karen Thompson, told Ms. Kowalski's parents about their lesbian relationship. Mr. Kowalski was named his daughter's guardian in an out-of-court agreement that allowed Ms. Thompson broad visiting rights to Ms. Kowalski, who was in a nursing home. In July 1985 Mr. Kowalski received unconditional guardianship and barred Ms. Thompson and other friends from any contact with his daughter. In September 1988, Ms. Kowalski was moved, by a court order, to a different nursing home for an evaluation of her competency, and there she was reunited with Ms. Thompson. The final determination of her competency, placement, and guardianship are still unsettled (*New York Times* 1989c).

Similar cases arise when one partner has AIDS. When the disease involves neurological impairments and dementia as an end-stage complication, the issue of a patient's competence is further clouded. Molly Cooke, a physician at San Francisco General Hospital, describes a typical case. A 27-year-old man with AIDS designated his lover as proxy and stated clearly that he did not want "heroics" when he reached the terminal stage of his illness. The physician understood him to mean that he refused intubation and mechanical ventilation. When the patient's parents arrived to visit him from out of town, they learned that he was gay at the same time that they learned he had AIDS. Angry and upset, they insisted that "everything be done" and threatened to sue the hospital. The lover withdrew as proxy and the physicians felt obliged to continue aggressive treatment. The patient died after 22 days on a respirator in the intensive care unit (Cooke 1986).

In another San Francisco case, a 32-year-old gay man with Kaposi's sarcoma had been abandoned as a child by his parents and was raised by a grandmother. She refused to care for him when she learned of his diagnosis. His siblings refused to visit him, and his parents wrote to tell him that God was punishing him for being gay. The patient designated his partner as his durable power of attorney for health care, and affirmed his refusal of intubation should he become incompetent. After his death, the patient's father insisted that the body be flown to the Midwest for burial, even though the patient had stated his desire for cremation and a local funeral. In this case the patient's wishes were honored, because of the durable power of attorney (Steinbrook et al. 1985).

In still another case, which reached the courts, Thomas Wirth, an AIDS patient at Bellevue Hospital in New York City, signed a living will refusing extraordinary treatment and naming a friend, John Evans, as guardian. The physicians challenged the directive, however, because it did not clearly specify which treatments were being refused. Evans took the case to court, but the court upheld the physicians. They argued that the particular condition that they were proposing to treat—a brain infection—was not by itself fatal. Mr. Wirth died soon after the decision.[1]

These cases illustrate common dilemmas but they are atypical in one respect: In each case the patient had clear preferences and had taken some steps to implement them. Unfortunately, as Cooke (1986, 345) points out, "many patients will be admitted to the hospital unable to express their wishes, without a previous documented discussion and without having appointed a proxy with durable power of attorney." If this is true among the predominately gay patient population of San Francisco, it is even more the case among the drug users and their sexual partners who now make up the majority of cases in New York City.

Kevin Kelly (1987), a psychiatrist at New York Hospital, has raised another possibility:

> Until now, the prevailing practice has been that, when a decision cannot be made by the patient or responsible others, physicians feel obliged to proceed as if the patient had given consent for all possible measures, but this epidemic may force us to reconsider this practice, and to substitute an alternative model in which the patient is assumed to have withheld consent unless it is specifically given.

Acknowledging that this model would sharply conflict with legal precedent, Kelly suggests that it would be applicable only when the patient is known to have an irreversibly terminal illness, his or her wishes cannot be determined, and there is no one else to make the decision. Such a model may hold considerable appeal for physicians, especially since

---

[1]*Evans v. Bellevue Hospital* (re Wirth), 16536 N.Y. Sup. (July 27, 1987).

some of the life-prolonging interventions, which are generally futile anyway, involve an additional, albeit small level of risk of HIV exposure to health care workers through needle sticks and blood splashes. It would, however, result in withholding care from a particular class of patients on the basis of their social status. The category of patients most likely to be affected would be the poor, probably minority, drug user, isolated from both family and friends. These patients would also be more likely to enter the health care system at a later stage of disease, thereby being more likely to have diminished competence. To deny care to such patients when care would be provided to similar patients who were fortunate enough to have social supports would be discriminatory.

Thus, AIDS is having an impact on treatment decisions. Physicians who regularly care for gay AIDS patients, as well as many patients themselves, are moving toward early, specific, and ongoing discussions about treatment, including its termination. The *AIDS Legal Guide* encourages persons with AIDS to "sign a Living Will if it represents their sentiments on the matter, because it serves as a communication of one's intent at a later time when one is no longer able to communicate" (Rubenfeld 1987, sec.9, p.4). The New York State law on "orders not to resuscitate," passed in April 1988, specifically included "a close friend" among those who may be designated to act as surrogate on behalf of the patient to acknowledge the rights of gay partners to participate in "do not resuscitate" (DNR) decisions[2] (Nancy Dubler, personal communication 1988). This trend clearly strengthens the force of advance directives in non-AIDS cases and sets an example for physician/patient communication for other life-threatening illnesses.

But autonomous decision making in matters of health care may be neither as important nor as easy to implement for patients from poor, minority backgrounds. A sense of fatalism, powerlessness, religious traditions, acquiescence to the wishes of others—whether they are family or physicians—all may work against patient self-determination. Intravenous drug users are not generally interested in talking about living wills and durable powers of attorney; they just want to be treated, hoping and praying for the best. Here too, AIDS will test boundaries, in this case those of personal autonomy and family control.

---

[2]New York State Public Health Law, Article 29-B (Orders not to resuscitate), L. 1987, ch. 818. Effective April 1, 1988.

AIDS may change the boundaries to include serious considerations of euthanasia or "assisted suicide," thus creating an enormous additional potential for conflict within families. AIDS may even test the validity of informed consent as the basis of medical decision making. At the very least it will require renewed attention to the importance of communication among and between patient, physician, and family. Physicians and hospital ethics committees may need special help in understanding, accepting, and dealing with nontraditional family members as participants in this process. When the appointed surrogate — for information or for decision making — does not bear the usual relationship to the patient, traditional norms of professional practice may be threatened.

Housing

All families need shelter, and nontraditional families have particular difficulties in obtaining and retaining housing, because of restrictive zoning ordinances and tenancy laws. Zoning laws established in the post-World-War-II building boom reflected the expectation that the typical family would consist of parents and children. Furthermore, zoning ordinances were intended to protect property values; deviations from the norm of the traditional family constellation are seen as economic threats. Such ordinances typically prohibit nonrelated individuals from sharing a single-family home. Thus, in addition to gay couples or young unmarried heterosexual couples, elderly couples who cannot afford to marry because their Social Security payments will be reduced may have difficulty in finding a place to live.

In Denver in May 1989, after considerable discussion, the city council voted to amend its 36-year-old ordinance and allow two adults unrelated by blood, marriage, or adoption to live in the same house. The new ordinance also eliminates a $20 room-and-board permit for an unrelated couple living together. The earlier prohibition affected mainly unmarried couples living together, as well as single parents who rent out rooms to tenants to help defray expenses (*New York Times* 1989d, 1989e). Councilwoman Mary de Groot applauded the ruling: "Zoning should be used for regulating land use and density, not relationships." An opponent of the change, Councilman Bill Roberts, who is black, saw the move, however, as threatening Afro-American family stability:

"The most stable environment in which to raise children is in a house with a mother and a father who have a commitment to each other."

New York's highest court, the State Court of Appeals, upheld a lower court that ruled that the town of Brookhaven's zoning law violated the state constitution by restricting the number of unrelated people who could live together as a "functionally equivalent family." The decision will make it easier for unrelated individuals to live together in areas previously restricted to single-family use (*New York Times* 1989f).

In 1974 the U.S. Supreme Court had, however, upheld a law in the village of Belle Terre, also in Long Island, that defined a family as people related by blood, marriage, or adoption, or not more than two unrelated people.[3] Recent amendments to the Federal Fair Housing Act,[4] extending governmental protections against housing discrimination to disabled people and families with children, may have a powerful impact on the rights of people with AIDS and their families to obtain housing.

In urban areas, a common problem arises when the person named on a lease dies and the surviving partner or family member claims the right to remain as a tenant in a rent-controlled or rent-stabilized apartment. The case of *Braschi v. Stahl Associates Company*[5] in New York City is the most significant legal challenge to the practice of limiting survivors' rights to traditional family members. Although the case involves a gay couple, the precedent it sets will be important for many people affected by the disease in low-income, minority communities, as well as for unmarried heterosexual couples and other nontraditional families. The situation is particularly dire for survivors who themselves are HIV-infected or have AIDS or who have responsibility for caring for another family member with AIDS. Eviction from an apartment upon the death of the primary tenant can lead to homelessness for the survivors.

Miguel Braschi lived with his life-partner Leslie Blanchard in Blanchard's rent-controlled New York City apartment for ten years, until Blanchard died of AIDS. Braschi, who was Blanchard's primary caregiver throughout his illness, was informed by the landlord that he was being evicted. The Supreme Court of New York County granted a pre-

---

[3]*Village of Belle Terre et al. v. Boraas et al.*, 416 U.S.1 (1974).
[4]P.L. 100–430 (September 13, 1988).
[5]*Braschi v. Stahl Associates Company*, 74 N.Y. 2d 201 (1989).

liminary injunction, halting the eviction. The judge found that, on the basis of the ten-year relationship, Braschi was a "family member" within the meaning of the rent control law, Section 56(d) of the New York City Rent, Rehabilitation and Eviction Regulations. This section provides that "family members who reside continuously for at least six months with the tenant of record, continue as rent-controlled tenants even after the tenant of record dies or vacates the premises."

The landlord appealed, and the appellate division unanimously reversed the decision. While it recognized that Braschi had proved that the relationship with the tenant had been "marked by love and fidelity for each other," it interpreted the rent control law "as only protecting surviving spouses and family members within traditional, legally recognized familial relationships." Braschi received permission for a direct appeal to the Court of Appeals, which decided in his favor in July 1989. Writing for the majority, Judge Titone said: "The term family . . . should not be rigidly restricted to those people who have formalized their relationship by obtaining, for instance, a marriage certificate or an adoption order. The intended protection against sudden eviction should not rest on fictitious legal distinctions or genetic history, but instead should find its foundation in the reality of family life." Further cases will undoubtedly seek to extend the ruling to rent-stabilized apartments and other types of housing, and some difficulties can also be expected in defining whether a particular couple meet the criteria for "family" set out in the decision — "two adult lifetime partners whose relationship is long-term and characterized by an emotional and financial commitment and interdependence."

Custody Decisions

Parents are normally responsible for the care and nurturing of their children. But when circumstances prevent one or both parents from fulfilling this obligation, courts determine who shall have custody of the child. The state's interest is in seeing that the child is protected, as much as possible, from the harmful effects of divorce, separation, or death. Traditionally, judges have wide latitude in determining a child's "best interests." Until recently the traditional presumption has favored, however, the biological mother. The *Baby M* case in New Jersey marked a deviation from this traditional course; the biological or "surrogate" mother, Mary Beth Whitehead, was defeated in her bid for custody by the biological father William Stern and the adoptive mother Elizabeth Stern. In general, courts are becoming much more responsive to paternal claims for custody.

Against this background, conflicts about custody of children related to AIDS or HIV infection arise in two broad contexts: visitation rights in separation and divorce cases, where one parent is lesbian or gay or is HIV-infected or has AIDS; and the placement of children following the death of a parent with AIDS.

As homosexuality has become more openly discussed and, arguably, more accepted in society, homosexual or bisexual parents have become more willing to seek custody of their children when a marriage or sexual relationship dissolves. And in general more courts have been willing to accept these nontraditional relationships. But to the already volatile atmosphere of a failed relationship, the question of HIV infection adds an explosive charge.

How will judges weigh HIV status in making custody decisions? A judge who might have been willing to grant custody to a gay parent may not be so amenable if he is misinformed about the possibilities of HIV transmission in a family setting. In the Indiana case of *Stewart v. Stewart*,[6] Mr. Stewart sought to regain visitation rights to his one-year-old daughter after his former wife refused to let him see her. Mrs. Stewart was addicted to drugs and alcohol, and had lost custody of her first two children before she met and married Mr. Stewart. A trial court held that Mr. Stewart could be denied all visitation rights to his daughter because he was HIV positive, although asymptomatic. An appeals court ruled, however, that HIV infection per se was not a reason to deny custody or visitation.

A New York court ruled, in *Jane and John Doe v. Richard Roe*,[7] that a father who had custody of his two children did not have to undergo HIV antibody testing as a condition of retaining custody, as the children's maternal grandparents had requested. The court in *Ann D. v. Raymond D.*[8] made a similar finding, ruling that "a positive test result may not automatically be a 'determinant factor' with respect to plaintiff's ability to be a custodial parent."

Courts in other jurisdictions, however, have restricted the visitation

---

[6] *Stewart v. Stewart*, 521 N.E. 2d 956 (Ind. Ct. App. 1988).
[7] *Jane and John Doe v. Richard Roe*, 526 N.Y. Sup. 718 (March 14, 1988).
[8] *Ann D. v. Raymond D.*, 528 N.Y. 2d 718 (1988).

rights of a parent with AIDS. For example, a New Jersey court ordered that a father with AIDS could not visit his child without supervision.[9]

Based on a review of the scientific and legal literature, Nancy Mahon (1988) concludes:

> A court's use of a parent's HIV infection as per se evidence of parental unfitness contravenes the best interests standard . . . unless judges perform a factually specific examination of how a particular parent's HIV infection affects a child, the child's best interests cannot be served.

Will future courts follow this standard? It will depend on judges' level of understanding and education. Hard cases, however, will inevitably arise, in which a parent's desire for custody must be weighed against the ability of that parent to provide appropriate care if he or she is seriously ill and likely to die or engaging in behavior like drug use that undermines the stability of the child's life.

A second category of custody case is arising as increasing numbers of mothers become ill with AIDS. These cases now occur where there are substantial numbers of infected and ill women, especially in New York, New Jersey, and Florida; as the epidemic progresses, they may be expected to arise elsewhere. The New York City Task Force estimates that "over the next few years a minimum of 60,000–70,000 children in New York City will lose at least one parent to AIDS. Of these, maybe 10,000 will lose both parents to the disease" (New York City AIDS Task Force 1988).

The surviving children, some of whom may be HIV-infected but many of whom are not, must be placed in someone's care. Whose should it be? The options for these children, the majority of them from poor minority families, are few and frequently bleak: placement with a member of the extended family who may be beset by the same social and economic problems as the natural mother; foster care, with its inherent impermanence; adoption, which is unlikely to be available for older children.

Frequently, decisions about custody are made by a dying mother; her wishes may conflict with those of surviving family members, the child, or the professional team caring for her. Sometimes a child may

---

[9] *Jordan v. Jordan*, FV 12-1357-84 (Middlesex County, N.J., Sup.).

wish to live with a relative whom the professionals consider ill-equipped for the responsibility but who may be the only biological relative. The legal options available to confer guardianship, such as testamentary provisions or deeds, are fraught with uncertainties (C. Zuckerman, personal communication 1988).

As family courts become overwhelmed with these cases (not just as a result of AIDS, but of drug, particularly crack, addiction as well), it is likely that the decisions will be based more on which party has the most effective legal representation and not on the ill-defined concept of "best interests of the child." In addition to effective representation for mothers, advocates for the children may be required to ensure that they do not become pawns in an intra- or interfamilial or agency/family dispute.

It is possible that courts' traditional preference for granting custody to biological parents, even those who have not demonstrated a high level of concern for their children, may collapse under the weight of the caseload of orphaned children and drug-addicted parents. The foster care systems in affected communities may also be unable to accommodate a huge number of children with multiple problems, because many of the potential foster parents may also be affected by the disease. If the foster care system collapses, it is possible that some children may be placed in states far from their communities of origin, rather like the Asian children brought to this country by adoptive parents. It is also possible that the very foundation of child placement since the Progressive Era—that children are better off in families than in institutions—may be re-examined. In New York City, however, group homes set up to accommodate "boarder babies" released from hospitals and awaiting foster care placement are understaffed, in disrepair, and violate health and safety regulations (*New York Times* 1989g).

In the future, custody decisions may, from necessity as much as principle, accommodate a wide variety of nontraditional family placements. With increased flexibility in these arrangements, it seems likely that most children could be placed in families. But some children—those hardest to place or those living in areas where families able and willing to accept them are in short supply—may have to live in institutions. Lois Forer (1988), a retired family court judge in Philadelphia who has seen at first hand the failures of both families and foster care, has already called for a return of orphanages. She says:

Public institutions are answerable to the public. They can be inspected regularly by public officials. Committees of private citizens can act as overseers and keep a careful eye on the operations of such orphanages. It is difficult and expensive for social workers to inspect at frequent intervals all foster homes.

The choice may come down to admittedly inadequate family placement and admittedly but differently inadequate institutional placement. A change in basic social work philosophy, which has favored families over institutions, would be profound and disturbing, but is not unthinkable.

The Formation of New Families

The process of change and adaptation is incomplete. Just as existing families continue to adjust to the exigencies of AIDS, the formation of new families may also be affected by law and changing custom. Individuals do not ordinarily make the commitment that defines "family" without considerable prior interaction with the potential partner. Families start out as relationships. If evidence for the impact of AIDS in the areas already described is scant, it is even more fragmentary the more one looks to the future for families. This final section is, therefore, largely speculative.

Some changes may reflect the epidemiology of AIDS. For example, in some minority communities, large numbers of men and women of childbearing age are HIV-infected. These communities place a high cultural value on reproduction; children are seen as proof of virility or femininity, sources of pleasure, links to the past, and hope for the future. How will HIV infection, and the consequent threat of the birth of HIV-infected babies, affect the formation of new relationships in these communities? Will a partner's HIV status be an important determinant? Will the post-AIDS society envisioned in Margaret Atwood's (1986) *The Handmaid's Tale*, in which healthy women serve as breeders, come to pass? It is not implausible that the wives of hemophiliacs or other men with HIV infection will choose artificial insemination rather than risk unprotected sex, HIV transmission to themselves, and infection of their fetuses. Nor is it far-fetched to think that some infected women would choose not to bear children themselves but would engage a surrogate for that purpose.

Even among groups where procreation is not a supreme value, HIV status may be influential in the formation of new relationships that might lead to procreation. Public policy and medical practice may play a significant role. The intent of mandatory premarital HIV screening (which was tried and abandoned in Louisiana and later in Illinois), as well as of less coercive efforts to encourage voluntary testing among couples about to be married or women considering pregnancy, is to discourage marriage and reproduction among HIV-infected partners. For example, two epidemiologists reviewing data about heterosexual transmission concluded that "societies may soon have to wrestle with many difficult questions, including the suitability of infected individuals for marriage and natural parenthood" (Haverkos and Edelman 1988). In challenging this "incautiously worded" comment, Ronald Bayer (1989) declared: "Both moral sensibilities and our constitutional tradition revolt at the notion that classes of adults—defined in terms of biologic factors—be barred from marriage." The authors replied: "We personally do not support criminalized marriage, criminalized childbirth, coerced abortion, or compulsory sterilization. . . . Nevertheless, . . . we can predict that as the pandemic widens and deepens in our society, increasingly powerful voices will be heard calling for such state-imposed restrictions" (Edelman and Haverkos 1989).

So far only one state (Utah) has passed a law invalidating marriages involving an HIV-infected partner. This law has not been tested. While the intent of the Utah law may be to protect traditional family norms, another source of opposition to sex involving HIV-infected partners comes from the Rajneesh religious communities, which reject exclusive, monogamous relationships. In their view, AIDS confirms their belief that AIDS is the result of sexual repression. One Rajneeshee explained: "What they [all those Christians and bourgeoisie] can't see is that the family is what drove all those people to rebel in the first place—to become homosexuals and junkies. So, returning to the family would only worsen the situation!" (Palmer 1989).

While organized opposition to marriage or sex involving an infected person may be limited, personal choices of sexual and especially marriage partners, only recently (and incompletely) freed from considerations of religion, race, and economic or social status, may be tempered by disease. Even though AIDS is becoming a chronic illness, the HIV-infected person has a shorter life span than a healthy person. Those involved in a sexual relationship, which includes the vast majority of married couples, must always be constrained by concerns about transmission. An attorney with hemophilia described a failed romance:

> Not long after I was diagnosed as carrying the virus, I began dating a bright, attractive woman. I wanted to kiss her—certainly no big thing under normal circumstances. But I felt I must first tell her about the virus. . . . On a rational basis, she grasped that kissing me would almost certainly not be dangerous. But AIDS has taken on an identity all its own. . . . It was a world of which she wanted no part. Recreational sex was not worth risking one's life for, she explained, and what was the point of developing strong emotions for someone who could not lead a normal sex and family life? (*New York Times Magazine* 1989a).

Disagreeing that life with HIV infection was inevitably asexual, the wife of a hemophiliac who died of AIDS nevertheless responded in a way that seemed to bear out the attorney's fears:

> I married my husband . . . after he was diagnosed with AIDS. It is true that we had a pre-existing relationship. However, it is also true that we had a romantic and sexual life after he was diagnosed. . . . I admit that the latter made me and my husband anxious, and that the anxiety could not be overcome completely (*New York Times Magazine* 1989b).

Although the stigma and discrimination surrounding the disease may diminish, they will not disappear. While existing relationships may survive and even be strengthened by knowledge of a partner's HIV infection, the formation of new relationships may well be deterred by the realities of the situation. On the other hand, there may be greater interest in, and social acceptance of, the legalization of marriages between homosexual partners (*New York Times* 1989h). The City of San Francisco's registry of "domestic partners" is a step toward legalization. Even in the absence of a formal mechanism, gay couples may announce their commitment in other ways. In New York City, Michael Feierstein, who works on AIDS programs in the Department of Health, and his lover, Luke Denobriga, a hairdresser, announced their plans to hold a "commitment ceremony" and to change their name to Mr. and Mr. Stanton (Luke's actual first name). In a memo to his colleagues, Mr. Feierstein said:

There is no mechanism in our society for gay people to publicly announce their relationships or "marriage." We're not permitted, by law, to marry. A recent trend in the Gay and Lesbian Community has been toward commitment ceremonies, wedding-like events for family and friends similar to those heterosexual people have been enjoying for centuries" (*Newsday* 1989b).

In this explication the differences between nontraditional and traditional families seem less important than their similarities. AIDS is both heightening the creation of nontraditional families and presenting special problems for them. AIDS threatens the intimacy and acceptance that ideally undergird family relationships, while at the same time making them all the more powerful and necessary.

References

Anderson, E.A. 1988. AIDS Public Policy: Implications for Families, *New England Journal of Public Policy* 4:411–27.

Atwood, M. 1986. *The Handmaid's Tale*. New York: Fawcett.

Bayer, R. 1989. The Suitability of HIV-positive Individuals for Marriage and Pregnancy. *Journal of the American Medical Association* 261:993.

Breo, D.L. 1988. Harlem Pediatrician's Concern: Fighting for Children with AIDS. *American Medical News* (October 21):3, 33.

Chicago Tribune. 1987. Obstacles for AIDS Victims: Hispanics Hampered by Poverty, Language Barrier, by J.L. Griffin. December 1.

Citizens Commission on AIDS. 1989. *The Crisis in AIDS Care: A Call to Action*. New York.

City of Los Angeles Task Force on Family Diversity. 1988. *Strengthening Families: A Model for Community Action*. Final Report.

Cohen, E.N. 1987. *Appointing a Proxy for Health-care Decisions: Analysis and Chart of State Laws*. New York: Society for the Right to Die.

Cooke, M. 1986. Ethical Issues in the Care of Patients with AIDS. *Quality Review Bulletin* 12:343–46.

Donzelot, J. 1979. *The Policing of Families*. New York: Pantheon.

Edelman, R., and H.W. Haverkos. 1989. The Suitability of HIV-positive Individuals for Marriage and Pregnancy. *Journal of the American Medical Association* 261:993.

Forer, L.G. 1988. Bring Back the Orphanage. *Washington Monthly* 20(3):17–24.

Frost, R. 1971 [1914]. *Poems*. New York: Washington Square Press.

Haverkos, H.W., and R. Edelman. 1988. The Epidemiology of AIDS among Heterosexuals. *Journal of the American Medical Association* 260:1922-29.

Kelly, K. 1987. AIDS and Ethics: An Overview. *General Hospital Psychiatry* 9:331-40.

Levitan, S.A., R.S. Belous, and F. Gallo. 1988. *What's Happening to the American Family?: Tensions, Hopes, Realities*. Rev. ed. Baltimore: Johns Hopkins University Press.

Lloyd, G.A. 1988. HIV-infection, AIDS, and Family Disruption. In *The Global Impact of AIDS*, ed. A.F. Fleming, New York: Alan R. Liss.

Mahon, N.B. 1988. Public Hysteria, Private Conflict: Child Custody and Visitation Disputes Involving an HIV-infected Parent. *New York University Law Review* 63:1092-1141.

Newsday. 1987. AIDS: Trouble in a Permissive Society, by A. Peracchio. November 10.

———. 1989a. AIDS Patients' Seder Held by Synagogue. April 18.

———. 1989b. And You Think Your Life is Complicated?, by J. Nachman. April 30.

New York City AIDS Task Force. 1988. *Models of Care Report*. New York.

New York Times. 1988. Mother of AIDS Victim Shares Her Story to Teach Others, by T. Morgan. November 25.

———. 1989a. Two Men Who Fought L.I. Abortion, by E. Schmitt. February 13.

———. 1989b. San Francisco Votes Legislation Recognizing Unmarried Partners. May 24.

———. 1989c. Woman's Hospital Visit Marks Gay Rights, by N. Broznan. February 8.

———. 1989d. Denver Zoning Fight Turns on Defining a Family. March 26.

———. 1989e. Denver Kills Law That Barred Homes with Unwed Couples. May 3.

———. 1989f. Court Upsets Long Island Zoning Law on Unrelated People in Home, by P.S. Gutis. March 24.

———. 1989g. Health Violations Cited at Child Group Homes, by S. Daley. May 20.

———. 1989h. Gay Marriages: Make Them Legal, by T.B. Stoddard. March 4.

New York Times Magazine. 1989a. A Life in Limbo, by P. Bayer. April 2.

———. 1989b. A Life in Limbo, by M.B. Ockey. April 23.

Palmer, S.J. 1989. AIDS as Metaphor, *Society* 26:44-50.

Rubenfeld, A.R. 1987. *AIDS Legal Guide*. 2nd ed. New York: Lambda Legal Defense and Education Fund.

Society for the Right to Die. 1987. *Handbook of Living Will Laws*. New York.

Sontag, S. 1986. The Way We Live Now. *New Yorker*.

Steinbrook, R., B. Lo., J. Tirpack, J.W. Dilley, and P.A. Volberding. 1985. The Ethical Dilemmas in Caring for Patients with the Acquired Immunodeficiency Syndrome. *Annals of Internal Medicine* 103:787-90.

Tiblier, K.B., G. Walker, and J. Rolland. 1989. Therapeutic Issues when

Working with Families of Persons with AIDS. In *AIDS and Families*, ed. E. Macklin, 81–128. Binghamton, N.Y.: Harrington Park.

Toffler, A. 1980. *The Third Wave*. New York: Bantam Books.

Tolstoy, L. 1981 [1877]. *Anna Karenina*. Tr. by J. Carmichael. New York: Bantam Books.

U.S. Bureau of the Census. 1981. *Marital Status and Living Arrangements: March 1980*. Washington.

———. 1988. *Households, Families, Marital Status and Living Arrangements: March 1988*. Advance report. Washington.

AIDS and the Prison System

NANCY NEVELOFF DUBLER and VICTOR W. SIDEL

C ORRECTIONAL INSTITUTIONS SERVE TO INCARCERATE offending individuals; to protect society from them (and them from society); to reform or rehabilitate them; or to exact what is viewed as just punishment. Prisons (for those convicted and sentenced to terms exceeding one year) and jails (for those awaiting trial or sentenced to short terms of a year or less) in the United States are not static: they change in ways that reflect the values, attitudes, and needs of the larger society. They change in response to who is remanded to them, in what numbers, and for which offenses; they change in response to the resources invested in them; and they change in response to their own internal culture. But, perhaps most important in our society, prisons and jails also respond and adapt to the process of judicial review and intervention.

Prisons are confining, not caring, institutions, and adapting to AIDS presents a fundamental dilemma. Their responses lay bare discrepancies between social expectations about the "correctional" function of prisons and the reality. Their efforts to cope with the disease exacerbate existing tensions over the jurisdiction of health care in prisons, and the disease necessarily blurs the boundaries between public health inside and outside the prison walls.

71

The Prison as an Environment
for Infection

Prisons are currently operating at overcapacity, and experts believe that excessive crowding will increase during the next decade—even as prison construction continues at a rapid rate.

> At midyear 1988, there were approximately one million people incarcerated in the United States—with almost three million more under the supervision of the criminal justice system through parole or probation services. This population has expanded 38 percent since 1984, and approximately one in 27 U.S. men now finds himself under some correctional supervision. Many state and local correctional systems are filled far beyond capacity. The National Council on Crime and Delinquency projects that the prison population will rise by over 68 percent by 1994, resulting in an additional 460,000 inmates (Shenson, Dubler, and Michaels 1990).

The startling growth in the number of prisons reflects both tougher police policies as part of the "war on drugs" and judicial determinate sentencing guidelines. There is now a "heightened likelihood that a serious offender will receive a prison sentence (as well as) a 113 percent increase in the number of adults arrested for drug trafficking or manufacturing" (*New York Times* 1990). In 1986, 54 percent of state prison inmates were under the influence of drugs or alcohol at the time of the offense (U.S. Bureau of Justice 1988; Potler 1988). Over 90 percent of the people who fill prisons and jails in the United States are men, and nearly half are African American. Almost all poor drug users rely on criminal behavior at some time to support their habits. Many ghetto residents, excluded from the job market, engage periodically in some aspect of the drug trade as one of the few means of employment open to them. Prisons are becoming, therefore, overwhelmingly crowded with people of color whose incarceration is associated in some way with drugs.

The increasing number of prisoners reflects the willingness of society to deal with drug use primarily through law-enforcement techniques. As expanded dragnets funnel drug users, dealers, and traffickers into the nation's prisons, there has been, not surprisingly, an explosion of drug use in prison, with all this implies for increased hostility, mistrust, and aggressive competition within correctional institutions. An underground prison drug economy increases danger for inmates and staff alike and encourages ever more repressive measures needed to sustain effective control. Drug use in the prisons will likely lead to the further corruption of officers, the emboldening of inmates, and increasing distrust between the two.

Individual health needs and public-health requirements in prisons have increased along with an expanded inmate population. "Prisons have now become the new tenements, overcrowded compounds, fertile and accommodating to disease" (Shenson, Dubler, and Michaels 1990). Accelerated urban decay, widespread illicit drug use, and poverty-associated epidemics — particularly tuberculosis and syphilis — have had a devastating impact on the health of prisoners. Prison medical services have been transformed into beleaguered outposts struggling to cope with near impossible demands (S. Zoloth, D. Michaels, and E. Bellin, Montefiore / Riker's Island Prison Health Service, personal communication 1990).

Rudimentary health care has been provided to confined inmates since the mid-nineteenth century. In England in 1784, social reformer Sir George Onesiphorus Paul instituted basic procedures for hygiene, not for the benefit of the prisoners, but rather to increase the "salutory humiliation" of prison life and to prevent the spread of epidemic disease beyond the prison walls to the general citizenry. The object was clear: ". . . the daily cleanups and hygienic inspections were intended not only to guard against disease, but also to express the State's power to order every feature of the institutional environment, no matter how minor" (Ignatieff 1978).

Health care in most correctional settings was woefully inadequate through the late 1960s when, following the revolt at Attica and the reports of civil-rights advocates who had experienced incarceration, citizens groups, civil-liberties organizations, and newly funded prisoners' rights attorneys began to investigate conditions of confinement. The conditions they found were shocking: prisoners performing surgery on fellow inmates; inmates left to die with wounds covered with maggots and encased in their own filth; and systems that separated sick and disabled inmates from medical caregivers by two locked sets of doors and no means of communication across them (Dubler and Sidel 1989).

In 1973, the U.S. Supreme Court decreed the end of the "hands off" doctrine that had insulated prisons and jails from judicial scrutiny and review.[1] This decision opened a floodgate of litigation challenging the lack of adequate health care and searching for a constitutional standard to measure the adequacy of health care in correctional facilities. In 1976, the Supreme Court's decision holding that the Eighth Amendment, which prohibits "cruel and unusual" punishment, stated that "deliberate indifference to the serious medical needs of inmates" constitutes a violation of an inmate's protected rights.

The courts went further: in January 1990 forty-one states (plus the District of Columbia, Puerto Rico, and the Virgin Islands) were ordered to reduce overcrowding and/or improve conditions of confinement, including provision of adequate medical care. In one case, a federal district court found a violation of the Eighth Amendment when an inmate died from heat prostration in an unventilated cell that reached 110°F, in a jail in which staff had not even had minimal medical training.[2] Testimony in the decision described a medical-care system in which intake physical examinations were performed in three minutes by a physician known to inmates as "Dr. No Touch"; infirmary rounds were done at the speed of one minute per patient and no inquiry was made into symptoms; and sick call was performed in a space so noisy that the doctor could not hear inmates' complaints. Nearly a decade and a half after the Supreme Court held that inmates have a constitutional right to health care,[3] lawsuits are still addressing basic problems of overcrowding, drug use, and inadequate medical treatment in facilities located in urban centers as well as isolated rural areas.

AIDS has flourished in this environment so ripe for the spread of infectious disease. And in a setting designed to confine, control, and punish, correctional health-service providers are called upon to diagnose, comfort, and treat. Tensions between correction officers and health staff are inevitable. The former see inmates as stripped of rights and liberties by the judicial process and condemned to a limited existence under properly humiliating circumstances. Health staff see the inmate as a patient with all the moral claims inherent in the doctor-patient relationship. Health-care providers must struggle constantly to avoid co-optation by the correctional ethic and to respect the autonomy

[1] *Procunier v. Martinez*, 416 U.S. 396 (1973).
[2] *Brock v. Warren County, Tennessee*, 713 F.Supp. 238 (E.D. Tenn., 1989).
[3] *Estelle v. Gamble*, 429 U.S. 97 (1976).

of patients as persons. AIDS has forced an uncomfortable alliance between the imperatives of care and those of punishment; correction officers and health providers must cooperate to provide decent health services and prevent the spread of AIDS.

The Prisoner with AIDS

The AIDS epidemic in prisons is most virulent in those states with high rates of seroprevalence among IV drug users (IVDUs). In 1988, the state of New York, for example, found a 17.4 percent HIV seroprevalence rate among prisoners tested anonymously as they entered the state prison system (Truman et al. 1989). Epidemiologists estimate that the number of prisoners with full-blown AIDS in the New York State Department of Corrections Services will rise from 800 at the end of 1989 to as many as 2,800 by the end of 1992 (Greifinger 1990). Many more are likely to be at earlier asymptomatic stages of the disease.

Among those dying of AIDS in the New York state correctional system, 95 percent had admitted to IV drug use (Potler 1988). AIDS patients die more quickly in prison than outside. In the New York state prison system, the median time between diagnosis and death is 159 days, compared with 318 days for nonprisoners. Many cases are not diagnosed until autopsy, indicating that opportunistic infections and AIDS in prisons are not recognized or treated adequately.

Inmates report that diagnosis of HIV infection or AIDS often leads to isolation and exclusion in the prison by other inmates and staff. Infected inmates are shunned, or attacked, or left to suffer alone with inadequate care. Those dying of AIDS mourn the loneliness of death away from family and support networks. One described himself as "an outcast in a society of outcasts" (*Newsday* 1988).

Some prison systems are segregating HIV-positive persons, but this procedure is controversial (even as it is in hospitals, schools, and other institutions). The Federal Bureau of Prisons, after testing all inmates and segregating the HIV positives for a few years, has discontinued this policy. The Colorado prison system in 1987 was among the first to segregate HIV seropositive male prisoners. The low number (under 25) permitted the prison to counteract overt discrimination by providing these inmates first access to desirable jobs and education programs. When the state of New York tried to segregate all known HIV seropositive inmates in one facility, the attempt was enjoined by the court as violating the inmates' rights to privacy, for segregation made their health status public. Moreover, the state had failed to provide the special services promised as a quid pro quo for segregation.[4] The court intimated that provision of additional health services might be sufficient for it to uphold segregation and the associated breach of confidentiality.

In *Harris v. Thigpen*, the Federal District Court in Alabama upheld segregation of HIV-positive persons and the mandatory testing of all entering inmates. The court found that segregation of all HIV-positive persons, as an administrative policy designed to prevent the spread of the disease, was constitutional because it was "reasonably related" to legitimate penological interests.[5]

AIDS may also be changing policies about experimentation on prisoners. Prisoners have been shielded from research, following analysis of the risks of research to human subjects, the historical abuse of prisoners, and an assumption that prisoners possess a diminished capacity to provide truly voluntary informed consent. But HIV infection is leading to a new consensus that prisoners should have access to Phase II and III clinical trials (those designed to determine efficacy in contrast to toxicity) as an option for care (Dubler and Sidel 1989; Dubler, Bergman, and Frankel 1990).

The ethical hazards of research in prisons remain, but the incentives for conducting research on the medical status of individual inmates has changed markedly, given the prevalence of HIV infection in inmate populations. Prisons may soon be the best site on which to study the progress of HIV infection in the IVDU community. Epidemiological research could be enormously helpful in understanding the progress of the epidemic. Prisoners themselves may want to volunteer for research as a way to get adequate health care or to obtain some other benefit. Some may volunteer for research, not for any tangible benefit but from a desire to be altruistic. Others may volunteer to relieve boredom, to enhance the prospect of ingratiation with the health-care or correctional administration, or to gain access to the power structure.

Indeed, AIDS has shown how far incarcerated people will go to press for leverage in the prison system. In *Harris v. Thigpen*, for example,

---

[4] *Doe v. Coughlin*, 71 N.Y. 2d 48, 518 N.E. 2d 536, 523 N.Y.S. 2d 782 (1987).
[5] *Harris v. Thigpen*, Civil Action No. 87V-1109-N, U.S. District Court for the Middle District of Alabama (Northern Division, decided January 8, 1990).

prisoners broke their traditionally united ranks against the correctional staff to take different stands on isolating HIV-positive inmates. One group of prisoners supported the plaintiffs — inmates opposing segregation — while another supported the defendants — correctional officers seeking to impose the policy. Highly sensationalized incidents of biting and blood throwing, moreover, suggest that a few desperate prisoners are using AIDS and fear of HIV transmission to intimidate staff and other inmates. These tactics, however, have evident limitations. At least one HIV-positive prisoner had years added to his sentence for biting a guard with the intention of infecting him. AIDS, in short, clarifies the narrow spectrum of opportunities prisoners have to gain advantage in the correctional system.

AIDS and Jurisdictional Tensions

Prisons as institutions suffer from contradictory U.S. Supreme Court decisions. The Court has expanded inmates' rights at the same time that it has granted ever broader discretion to prison administrators. It is well settled that prisoners maintain those civil rights that are not fundamentally incompatible with a prisoner's status or with the legitimate objectives of incarceration. It is also clear that prisoners retain some fundamental rights of personal privacy. The extent of prisoners' rights and the validity of administrative orders that impinge on those rights, however, are judged by whether the regulation is "reasonably related to legitimate penological interest."[6] Issues of mandatory testing, involuntary screening, segregation of HIV-positive persons, and perhaps even adequate and appropriate medical care will all be held to this "reasonableness" standard in scrutiny by the federal district courts. In prison health care, as in no other sphere of American life, the tension between the right to care and the duty to punish appears as a modern morality play.

This drama involves a confrontation with the major myths of prison life — that consensual same-gender sex and IV drug use do not exist in prisons. Both assertions are incorrect. High-risk behaviors do exist in the prisons; "prison officials, staff, and prisoners spoke quite candidly about the occurrence of IV drug use and anal intercourse inside the pri-

---

[6] *Turner v. Safley*, 107 S.Ct. 2254 (1987).

sons" (Potler 1988). One inmate explained that shooting up in the yard was particularly hazardous because all injectors shared needles. He explained that IV drug use was the most widespread high-risk practice, followed by homosexual intercourse and tattooing (Potler 1988). But corrections officials resist distributing bleach, fearing its use as a weapon against inmates and guards (Hornblum 1988).

They also resist the use of condoms. Sex between inmates is a fact of prison life. "According to the NPP [National Prison Project], consensual sex is the most prevalent. Almost as common is coerced sex, in which sexual favors are traded for protection from assault or for other benefits. Finally, rape takes place in nearly every American prison and jail, although precise figures are difficult to obtain" (Vaid 1987). Yet, because of deep-seated needs to deny the existence of sexual relationships in prison, inmates are exposed to unprotected transmission in prison. According to a report by lawyers with Prisoner's Legal Services, about 25 percent of state prison inmates in New York are sexually active. Despite this the Commissioner of Corrections stated: "I don't see the logic of providing inmates with the means to engage in activity I just told them was prohibited" (*Newsday* 1988).

The relationship between inmates and correctional staffs, like the relationships among inmates, is often no less brutal and rigid. It is structured by force, power, and intimidation, not logic or intellectual reasoning. Providing condoms is a constant challenge to the balance of power among all personnel in correctional institutions, to the rules prohibiting sexual relationships, and to the fiction that no fraternal and supportive relationships exist among inmates.

Persistent myths, often based on jurisdictional and power struggles, obstruct effective education about HIV infection. Acknowledging prevalent behaviors will expose the inadequate control of correctional administrators over consenting and nonconsenting sexual behavior, the ineffectiveness of drug interdiction programs, and the corruption and co-optation of staff. Correctional authority is legitimated by the criminal justice system; a few officers can control hundreds of inmates only if the myth of supremacy is accepted. The existence of intramural criminal and interdicted behaviors undermines the myth of control and therefore actual control as well.

In this context, correctional and public-health authorities must devise effective strategies for AIDS education — not only for life in prison, but also for protection of self and others upon release. These necessarily involve both professionals and inmates—the former to assure the accuracy and credibility of information; the latter to assure inmate trust, to guarantee access to all factions in the prison, and to encourage later reinforcement of the educational message. Yet, this prescription for effective education challenges some basic tenets of prison administration: to exclude outsiders (that is, professionals) who are not subject to correctional authority and, more important, never to permit the empowerment of inmates.

Inmate involvement in education and peer counseling, simply put, is a form of empowerment. It also implies the continued existence of prohibited actions. Prison officials interested in disseminating risk-reduction or safe-sex information have not reckoned with inmates' distrust of written documents, however. Many prisoners, including those with limited literacy skills, believe such documents might be incriminating. Although the Commissioner of Corrections for New York State averred three years ago "that every single inmate and every single staff member has gotten a book, and it's called '100 Questions and Answers About AIDS,' and it is available in Spanish and English," the distribution of the material may not have had the effect of reducing health risks—or empowering inmates through educational means (*Newsday* 1988).

The treatment of HIV infection in prisons is also likely to reveal a profound irony in the system of medical care in America. Inmates may have less than adequate medical care but they increasingly have more access to care than many other inner-city populations.

> They are the only group with the constitutional right to care. . . .
> Jails and prisons already represent a primary source of health care for poor and minority Americans, since a significant number of inner-city residents pass through the corrections system every year (Shenson, Dubler, and Michaels 1990).

The desire for continued incarceration in order to obtain needed treatment echoes the theme of the 1904 short story by O. Henry. The central character, a homeless man, attempts at the start of winter to have himself arrested in order to be sentenced to three months in the New York City jail on Blackwell's Island.

> [T]he Island loomed big and timely in Soapy's mind. He scorned the provisions made in the name of charity for the city's dependents.

In Soapy's opinion the Law was more benign than Philanthropy. . . .
[T]o one of Soapy's proud spirit the gifts of charity are encumbered.
If not in coin you must pay in humiliation of spirit for every benefit
received at the hands of philanthropy. . . . [I]t is better to be a
guest of the law, which, though conducted by rules, does not meddle
unduly with a gentleman's private affairs (O. Henry [1904] 1948).

Although O. Henry's "Baghdad-on-the-Subway" has surely changed
since 1904, and most of its tens of thousands of homeless people would
now prefer the degradation and risk of a city "shelter" to the degradation and risk of the Riker's Island jail, being a "guest of the law" may
be seen by some seriously ill victims of AIDS as preferable to seeking
largely unavailable charity care on the outside.

Indeed, HIV-infected inmates both from the Riker's Island jail and
from New York state facilities have been refusing parole; their reason is
the fear that they would not have continued access to treatment with
AZT once on the outside. The fear is neither unrealistic nor unjusti-
fied. New York city ambulatory clinics are seriously overcrowded, with
many months of waiting required to secure an appointment. Despite
the barrenness and tyranny of prison, even in a state system recently
charged with constitutionally inadequate AIDS care, the access is more
secure than in the "free" world.

Yet, a system designed and sanctioned by society to punish and control cannot turn into a system of caring. In a prison, sickness does not
redefine the moral and legal status of a criminal. There are also practical constraints on the role of prisons in dealing with disease. AIDS is
an acute illness and a chronic disease. A sufferer may have both raging
fevers and chronic incontinence. Prison guards have neither the personal relationships nor the professional skills to diaper a dying patient.
Nor is it acceptable to bring family or other support groups into the
therapeutic regimen of the prison.

Prisons will soon face the need to provide current guards with skills
in long-term care, or hire staff with such capabilities. New York, which
houses more prisoners with HIV infection than any other state, estimates that it will spend an extra $29 million in 1992 on contract ser-
vices for acute care if it has not created at least 151 long-term-care beds
by that point (Greifinger 1990). If these plans are not implemented,
two choices remain: to place inmates in community acute-care or long-
term-care facilities, or to keep them in the prison where other pris-

oners, only slightly less sick, will care for them. Prisons will become the new leper colonies segregated from society, where the infected are left to sicken and die.

Prison Culture and the Community beyond the Walls

The system of corrections is designed to segregate, confine, and punish; the system of medicine, to comfort and care. Since the 1976 Supreme Court decision determining that inmates have a constitutional right to care, these cultures have lived in an uneasy relationship. This precarious standoff is threatened by overcrowding, the importation of street drugs into prisons, and by AIDS. Given the demands of illness, guards will need to show concern rather than contempt for their charges. This change in attitudes is unlikely to happen to a sufficient degree to prevent prisons, in states with a high HIV seroprevalence among its drug users, from becoming grotesque containers for cries of suffering and lonely death.

The culture of prisons and jails is dominated by correction officers, who have, at least in theory, total control over inmates. Health-care providers are the only independent, autonomous, noncorrectional staff members regularly tolerated by a prison culture that abhors outsiders. Health workers must continually negotiate for adequate access to inmates for sick call, follow-up, consultant, and emergency-care visits. In prison only corrections controls the keys. Providers and inmates are subject to lock-downs and other security fiats.

Whether an institution's culture can accommodate to AIDS may reflect its degree of sympathy and flexibility: both are absent in the American correctional system. Correctional culture is rigid, hierarchical, and, occasionally, brutal—poor preparation for care of the acute and chronically ill. Nor does society want felons, especially those convicted of drug-related crimes, abroad in the land. Early release and medical furlough for AIDS patients are not popular programs with the public or legislators. We wedge ever more inmates into inadequate facilities as expansion of prisons and jails cannot keep pace with more active police and law-enforcement strategies for lock-up. Thus, prisons and jails are virtually certain to confine escalating numbers of HIV-infected individuals. The prognosis for the health of incarcerated people with HIV infection, and increasingly for incarcerated people with AIDS, is poor. Much will depend on the willingness of the federal courts to enforce the constitutional standard and impose caring policies on systems turned even more repressive by the crowding pressures that reflect societal consensus on drug and crime control.

The figures on HIV infection suggest that prisons are about to become hospital conduits and nursing homes if planning and funding are adequate, or charnel houses, if they are not (Dubler, Bergmann, and Frankel 1990). The constitutionally protected right to care, which is not "deliberately indifferent," will require provision of AZT (or possibly other drugs in the near future) for asymptomatic infection among those with appropriately low T-cell counts. No such right exists outside of prisons. Will the public abide such a "pro-inmate" policy? Will the courts enforce the previously settled law or retreat from vigorous enforcement? Will inmates who received treatment on the inside, and despair of access elsewhere, refuse parole? And will people seek arrest in order to gain access to care?

As prisons in areas of high seroprevalence seek sufficient numbers of acute and long-term-care beds, they will compete with the community for these scarce resources. The health needs of prison society will not be contained behind razor wire and concrete walls. Prison walls effectively restrain criminals only for short time spans; they neither delimit nor contain the public-health challenges of infectious disease. How we care for the incarcerated will have a direct effect on needed clinical and public-health services in the community. This will be increasingly the case as federal judges order release of inmates to alleviate overcrowding. Policies for furlough and parole, encouraged by overcrowding, shuttle prisoners between their cells and society, breaking the barriers between public health inside and outside the prison.

AIDS thus raises the question of whether correctional authorities alone have a controlling stake in the prisons or whether public-health authorities have legitimate aegis as well. Conventional divisions of governmental authority preclude this cooperation, and the culture of corrections is harshly resistant to change. Nevertheless, the data demonstrate beyond any doubt the need for systematic public-health interventions in prison.

References

Dubler, N.N., C.M. Bergman, and M.E. Frankel. 1990. Management of HIV Infection in New York State Prisons. *Columbia Human Rights Law Review* 21(2):363–400.

Dubler, N.N., and V.W. Sidel. 1989. On Research on HIV Infection and AIDS in Correctional Institutions. *Milbank Quarterly* 67:171–207.

Greenspan, J. 1988. NPP Gathers Statistics on AIDS in Prison. *Journal of the National Prison Project* 16:5–9.

Greifinger, R.B. 1990. Testimony to a Joint Hearing — Assembly Committee on Crime and Corrections and Health. January 17, Albany, New York.

Hornblum, A. 1988. The Condom Wars — Should America's Jails/Prisons Distribute Condoms? *American Jail.* Fall:23–27.

Ignatieff, M. 1978. *A Just Measure of Pain: The Penitentiary in the Industrial Revolution 1750–1850.* New York: Columbia University Press.

Newsday. 1988. Outcasts among Inmates, by Ron Howell. May 1.

New York Times. 1990. Better Mousetrap for the 1990's: It's a Prison Cell, by M. Winerip. June 15.

O. Henry (William Sydney Porter). 1904. The Cop and the Anthem. In *The Four Million.* New York: Doubleday and Company. (Reprinted in 1948 in *The Pocket Book of O. Henry Stories*, ed. H. Hansen, 14–20. New York: Simon and Schuster.)

Potler, C. 1988. *AIDS in Prison: A Crisis in New York State Corrections.* New York: Correctional Association of New York.

Shenson, D., N.N. Dubler, and D. Michaels. 1990. Jails and Prisons: The New Asylums. *American Journal of Public Health* 80:655–56.

Truman, B., D. Morse, J. Mikl, S. Lehman, R. Stevens, A. Forte, and A. Broaddus. 1989. HIV Seroprevalence Risk Factors among Prison Inmates Entering New York State Prisons. Abstract no. 4207 at the 4th International AIDS Conference, Stockholm. In *AIDS in New York State through 1988.* New York: New York State Department of Health.

U.S. Bureau of Justice. 1988. Profile of State Prison Inmates 1986. *Bureau of Justice Statistics.* NCJ-109926. Washington.

Vaid, U. 1987. *AIDS, Prisons, and the Law: A Guide for the Public*, ed. H.L. Dalton et al. New Haven: Yale University Press.

New Rules for New Drugs
The Challenge of AIDS to the Regulatory Process

HAROLD EDGAR and DAVID J. ROTHMAN

T HE AIDS EPIDEMIC, SUDDENLY AND SYSTEMATICALLY, is transforming American attitudes and practices about the regulation and use of drugs. In the 1970s, as psychiatrist Gerald Klerman (1974) astutely observed, Americans were pharmacological Calvinists and psychotropic hedonists, that is, ever so cautious and sparing about the drugs they took in the pursuit of health, and ever so open and daring about the drugs they took in the pursuit of pleasure. This orientation had rather odd effects not only on personal behavior (a reluctance to go on an antibiotic, no reluctance to try the newest sensation-expanding compound) but also on the direction of public policy. With a minimum of intellectual discomfort liberals simultaneously advocated that the government keep its regulatory hands off pleasure drugs (for example, legalize marijuana and heroin) and expand the authority of the Food and Drug Administration (FDA) so that, as we shall see, drugs like thalidomide would be kept off the market. Now, in the tide of the AIDS epidemic in the 1980s, these attitudes are being reversed. In the case of AIDS, the response is pharmacological hedonism — a willingness to try any drug with the whisper of a chance to halt the deadly progress of the infection — and there may be an insurgent psychotropic Calvinism — a mounting insistence on the fact that drugs can kill, indeed that pleasure (including sexual pleasure) is dangerous. And once again, these attitudes are restructuring policy. They encourage, at one and the same time, a war on drugs and a war on the FDA and other regulatory bodies — like the institutional review boards (IRBs) — that stand between the consumer and the drug manufacturer. In the course of this chapter, we will be focusing on the pharmacological side of this dualism, leaving to others to ponder the changes that AIDS may be bringing to psychotropic (and sexual) hedonism. The transformation in the pharmacological arena is of such critical dimensions as to well warrant full attention.

The Drug Control Model

The regulatory system that underlay the pharmacological Calvinism of the 1960s and 1970s was born of scandal. The enlarged authority of the Food and Drug Administration and the creation of the institutional review boards were both the result of widely perceived abuses on the part of drug manufacturers and biomedical researchers. It appeared as though the greed of the one and the ambition of the other was so unbounded that government had to intervene to protect the consumer/human subject. As against the dangers of a hands-off policy, the exercise of governmental paternalism seemed altogether justified.

The transforming moment in the history of drug regulation was 1962. Senator Estes Kefauver was winding up a long and only modestly successful campaign to regulate drug prices by demonstrating that the companies were reaping unconscionably huge profits. The companies' justifications notwithstanding, including considerable investment in new drug research and development, Kefauver insisted that the consumers were bearing an unfair burden (*Congressional Record* 1962a). But however impressive the testimony that he elicited, no changes in the law seemed likely to emerge from the hearings, at least until the thalidomide story broke. This drug, widely prescribed in Europe, was in the process of being evaluated for safety by the FDA. One official, Frances Kelsey, concerned by reports of peripheral neuropathy, delayed approval, and in the interim the link between thalidomide and birth defects (typically, warped limbs) became apparent. Kelsey later received the highest award for government service from President Kennedy (Lasagna 1989). Although a major catastrophe had been averted, some 20,000 Americans, of whom 3,750 were of child-bearing age and 624 were reported as pregnant, had already taken thalidomide on an "experimental" basis. These experiments were more part of drug company marketing efforts to persuade physicians to use the drug than bona fide efforts to test it. To make matters worse, the precise number of recipients was unknown and their identification incomplete, mostly because the companies and the prescribing physicians who were conducting the trials kept very sloppy records.

Kefauver took full advantage of the incident and the harsh light it shed on drug company practices to clinch the case for greater regulation. In fact, his case now became so compelling that the proposed legislation passed both the House and Senate unanimously (*Congressional Record* 1962a). Yet as often happens, the scope of the response far exceeded the nightmare case that provoked it. The Food, Drug, and Cosmetic Act (FDCA) changed drug-approval procedures from premarket notification to premarket approval. Before 1962 new drugs could be marketed after the pharmaceutical sponsor submitted safety data unless the FDA reviewed the data and said no; after 1962 the FDA had affirmatively to say yes, thus giving FDA staff reviewers and the advisory committees more responsibility for the decisions. Congress also required the FDA to evaluate drugs not only for safety (an authority it held since 1938) but for efficacy as well—even though efficacy was not an issue in the case of thalidomide (Lasagna 1989).[1]

The entire episode demonstrates how powerful the symbolic role of a nightmare case can be in the implementation of public policy. Sustaining the drug regulatory enterprise between 1962 and the AIDS crisis was the figure of an heroic Frances Kelsey, single-handedly saving Americans from tragedy by saying no to a drug manufacturer. The message was clear: those who exercise caution reap rewards; there were no prizes for government employees who said yes to a drug, no matter how effective it turned out to be. Moreover, this message was one to which the FDA staff was especially receptive, for those recruited to these positions, at salaries substantially below those in the private sector, were very likely to arrive with a sense of mission about consumer protection. Thus, it is not surprising that the FDA defined its goals after 1962 in terms of minimizing risk. Its purpose was to assure the safety of marketed products, leaving it to others like the National Institutes of Health (NIH), to worry about curing disease. The FDA, in

---

[1] 21 *U.S. Code* sect. 355(b) as amended by P. L. 87-781, sect. 102(b) (1962).

brief, had every incentive to avoid what statisticians call type 1 errors even at the price of type 2 errors of greater magnitude. Better to err on the side of safety, even if it meant keeping an effective drug off the market for a longer period.

Controls on Human Experiments

The development of regulatory authority over human experiments follows a similar and overlapping course. In the hearings and debates on the Kefauver bill, the senators learned, to the amazement of at least some, that patients who received experimental drugs in these preliminary trials did not always know that they were participants in an experiment and that the safety of the drug had not been established. New York's Senator Jacob Javits, profoundly disturbed by this finding, proposed an amendment to the Kefauver bill which would have compelled the Secretary of Health, Education, and Welfare to write regulations that "no such drug may be administered to any human being in any clinical investigation unless that human being has been appropriately advised that such drug has not been determined to be safe in use for human beings." As Javits explained: "I feel deeply that some risks must be assumed. . . . [Nevertheless,] experimentation must not be conducted in a blind way, without people giving their consent. . . . Where is the dignity, the responsibility, and the freedom of the individual?" But Javits's colleagues were unwilling to accept his proposal. In this early moment in the history of public policy and bioethical issues, they conflated experimentation with therapy and the investigator with the physician. They believed, for example, that requiring physicians to inform a patient about an experimental drug would also compel them to inform a patient about a diagnosis that was fatal (in 1962 an unthinkable principle), for it might happen that to get the patient to take the new drug the doctor would have to tell him that he was suffering from a life-threatening illness. With a "strict, mandatory, prenotification requirement," argued Florida's Senator Carroll, "we might prevent the doctor from helping his patients in times of extreme emergency" (*Congressional Record* 1962b). In effect, there seemed little reason to glove the hand of the researcher or deny patients/subjects the miracles of the laboratory.

But soon, once again as the result of scandals and whistle-blowers, this reluctance disappeared and the researcher became the object of widespread suspicion. The transforming moment was Henry Beecher's (1966) article in the *New England Journal of Medicine* on the ethics of human experimentation. At its heart were capsule descriptions of twenty-two examples of investigators who risked "the health or the life of their subjects" without informing them of the dangers or obtaining their permission. Example 2 constituted the purposeful withholding of penicillin from servicemen with streptococcal infections in order to study alternative means for preventing complications. The men were totally unaware of the fact that they were part of an experiment, let alone at risk of contracting rheumatic fever, which twenty-five of them did. Example 16 involved the feeding of live hepatitis viruses to residents of Willowbrook, a state institution for the retarded, in order to study the etiology of the disease and attempt to create a protective vaccine against it. In example 17, physicians injected live cancer cells into twenty-two elderly and senile hospitalized patients without telling them that the cells were cancerous, in order to study the body's immunological responses. Example 19 described how researchers inserted a special needle into the left atrium of the heart of subjects, some with cardiac disease, others normal, in order to study the functioning of the heart (Beecher 1966; Rothman 1987).

Beecher's most significant, and appropriately most controversial, conclusion was that "unethical or questionably ethical procedures are not uncommon" among researchers, that a disregard for the rights of human subjects was widespread. The twenty-two cases, he declared, had been too easy to compile; an earlier and longer draft of the article had a total of 50, which had to be winnowed down for publication (Beecher 1966).

The *New England Journal of Medicine* article captured an extraordinary amount of public attention. Accounts of Beecher's piece appeared in the leading newspapers and weeklies, and dismay was mixed with incredulousness as reporters, readers, and public officials alike wondered what led respectable scientists to commit such acts (Faden and Beauchamp 1986, chaps. 3–4). The impact was even more noticeable at the National Institutes of Health, the major funding agency of biomedical research. Dependent upon congressional funding and good will for its budget, the NIH had scrupulously to consider the implications of the exposés for its own operation. At least one congressman had written the NIH to inquire how it intended to respond to Beecher's cases, and its associate director hastened to assure him that the findings "as might be expected have aroused considerable interest, alarm, and apprehension," and that "constructive steps have already been taken to prevent such occurrences in research supported by the Public Health Service" (PHS) (Sherman 1966).

The congressman's letter was only the most visible sign of the NIH's vulnerability (or sensitivity) to political and legal pressure. Any Washington official who hoped to survive in office understood the need to react defensively, to have a policy on hand, so that when criticism mounted he would be able to say that, yes, a problem had existed, but procedures were already in place to resolve it. The NIH director, James Shannon, readily conceded that one of his responsibilities, even if only a minor one, was "keeping the government out of trouble." And his advisers concurred: it would be nothing less than suicidal to believe that "what a scientist does within his own institution is of no concern to the PHS" (Frankel 1973, 23). An ad hoc group appointed by Shannon to consider NIH policies reported back that if cases involving researchers' disregard of subjects' welfare came to court, the service "would look pretty bad by not having any system or any procedure whereby we could be even aware of whether there was a problem of this kind being created by the use of our funds" (Frankel 1973, 31).

The result of all of these elements was the creation of a collective mechanism whereby individual researchers had to obtain the approval of their peers—and of at least some representatives of the wider community—before they could conduct experiments that put humans at risk. By the mid-1970s, the NIH (and the Public Health Service) had in place a system whereby every institution that received their research funds had to organize an institutional review board to pass on each protocol. The IRB's principal assignment was to insure that the risks to the research subject did not outweigh the benefits, and that the subject had been informed of all the significant aspects of the research (including the right to withdraw from the experiment at any time), and had voluntarily consented to participate. Along with the IRB regulations came a series of specific rules and proposals that sought to protect the most vulnerable classes of subjects, that is, the once competent and the never competent (the institutionalized mentally ill and retarded, children, and the elderly) and prisoners. These groups had been the subjects in a majority of the protocols in Beecher's roster of dishonor, and the new regulations made it difficult, at times impossible, to use them in experimentation. Once the NIH–PHS system was developed, the FDA came aboard, requiring that protocols testing drugs on humans also secure approval from the IRBs (*Federal Register* 1971).

Thus, overlapping regulatory systems were established on the dual premises that drug manufacturers were unreliable, motivated more by profits than concern for the consumer, and researchers were untrustworthy, motivated more by ambition than by concern for the patient. Put another way, the definition of the problem that underlay the government response, the cases that came to mind when regulations were written, were of thalidomide and Willowbrook, the former justifying the apparatus of the FDA, the latter, the apparatus of the IRB.

Following this orientation, these two regulatory systems shared a number of special characteristics:

First, the FDA and the IRBs both relied heavily on a standard of "sound science," hopeful that its postulates would rein in the ambitions of pharmaceutical companies and individual investigators. In the ethics of human experimentation, this precept had been announced by judges in rule 5 of the Nuremberg Code: "The experiment should be so designed and based on the results of animal experimentation and a knowledge of the natural history of the disease or other problems under study that the anticipated results will justify the performance of the experiment" (*Trials of War Criminals before the Nuremberg Military Tribunals* 1949, vol. 2, pp. 181–82). The rule's contemporary embodiment became the federal regulation declaring that IRBs must review research to assure that procedures are consistent with "sound research design" and do not unnecessarily expose subjects to risk. The IRBs must also assure that "risks to subjects are reasonable in relation to anticipated benefits."[2] Thus, bad science is unethical science. Yet, the tension between the norms of pure science – which relies heavily on the individual investigator's skepticism about conventional wisdom – and the authority of regulatory bodies, including nonscientists, to decide what constitutes good science went unnoticed, at least outside the corridors of research institutions.

Similarly, the role of "sound science" became central to the FDA's administration of the drug control model even as it had a paradoxical relation to the real world of medical practice. The law prohibits anyone

---

[2] 45 *Code of Federal Regulations* sect. 46.111(a)(2) (1988).

from introducing into commerce a "new drug" unless the drug is covered by an approved "new drug application"(NDA).[3] The FDA can approve such an NDA only if the drug is safe and if substantial evidence from adequate and well-controlled trials demonstrates that the drug is effective.[4] Safety and efficacy are measured in relation to the drug's utility in treating the particular diseases delineated in the drug's proposed labeling. The labeling becomes, in effect, an FDA-approved indication for the drug's use. During the 1960s and 1970s, the FDA demanded that drug manufacturers prove drug efficacy by multiple controlled clinical trials. Indeed, insisting on strict "scientific proof" of efficacy proved to be the vehicle by which the FDA accomplished the burdensome task, imposed on it by the 1962 Kefauver amendments, of reviewing the thousands of "new drugs" that had reached the market under NDAs from 1938 and 1962, when safety alone was the test; it revoked permission to market after a group of experts had determined that scientific proof of "efficacy" was lacking. By taking the position that manufacturers were not even entitled to a hearing unless there was evidence of efficacy derived from controlled clinical trials, the FDA avoided the necessity of time-consuming administrative hearings for hundreds of drugs. At such hearings doctors could have been expected to testify about all the patients a drug had helped in the course of their practices, and the pharmaceutical companies could claim this evidence "proved" drug efficacy. Such anecdotes are not evidence, the FDA ruled; data are not the plural of anecdote. The administrative task was accomplished, therefore, by delegitimating uncontrolled physician experience as a basis for permissive regulatory action. The law required scientific proof, and science required that drug efficacy be established through very exact and well-defined methods.[5]

However, neither science nor law controls what doctors do once the drug is on the market. Physicians can prescribe the drug for whatever purposes and in whatever doses they wish, subject only to whatever constraints are imposed by, for example, fear of malpractice suits or hospital pharmacy controls. The FDCA regulates commerce, not the practice of medicine. It is common, therefore, for drugs to be used for

---

[3]21 *U.S. Code Annotated* sect. 355(a) (West Supp. 1989).
[4]21 *U.S. Code Annotated* sect. 355(d) (West Supp. 1989).
[5]*Weinberger v. Hynson, Wescott and Dunning, Inc.* 412 U.S. 609, 612 (1973).

a much wider range of indications than "scientific evidence" supports. Physicians do their own "cost-benefit" analysis of new drugs once the compounds reach their hands, exercising the very type of professional discretion which, after 1962, was no longer the standard for gaining FDA drug approval. Thus, the insistence on scientific standards made securing an NDA an even greater economic prize, bringing rewards for successful drug innovation that even Kefauver could not have imagined. Obtaining an NDA gave the pharmaceutical companies a market not only for the listed indications, but, through physician discretion, a market, often much broader, for unlisted indications. More, obtaining an NDA may deter a competitor's entry with a different drug, unless the competitor is willing to incur heavy research and testing costs while facing a smaller market and is ready to run the risk that the FDA may not judge a second drug "safe" unless it has some advantage over the one already marketed.

Second, the new regulatory system assumed that being a research subject was a burden that should be distributed as equitably as possible. The premise was that human subjects were at risk, that taking part in an experiment was a sacrifice, and that sacrifice should be made by all, not just the helpless in society. So consent forms originally composed in English had to be translated into Spanish if the population to be recruited was heavily Hispanic, and if the form was not translated, for whatever reason, these subjects were not to be used.

Third, the system was prepared to make the trade-off of slower medical advances in return for better monitored ones. In the context of human experiments, the price was largely unacknowledged. Not only were the financial costs of the monitoring hidden in overhead and indirect cost allocations afforded to the research institution, but the possible social costs in slowing down or discouraging an individual investigator were very difficult to quantify or aggregate. In the context of drug review, however, the FDA's oversight did come in for withering attacks from both the pharmaceutical industry and a number of academicians. Their central complaint was that it cost too much and took too long to secure approval of a new drug. These critics posited a "drug lag," and argued that the incredible increase in the average length of time and costs in securing marketing approval for a new drug — from a couple of years and a few million dollars in 1960 before the Kefauver amendments to an average of ten years and nearly $100 million in the 1970s — undercut company incentives. (*Inside R&D* [1990] has updated the time for securing approval to 12 years, at a cost of $231 million.) The reduction explained the sharp drop in introduction of "new chemical entities" for pharmaceutical use. A variant on the drug-lag theme was that useful drugs first reached the market in Europe, because European nations' standards were more realistic, meaning that United States citizens received second-best care while the FDA procrastinated about possible side effects. Perhaps most poignantly, regulatory costs created therapeutic orphans, persons whose diseases or situations were sufficiently rare that it simply did not pay to produce therapies directed to them, even if one had a therapy that probably worked (Kaitin et al. 1989; Wardell 1973).

This is not the place to evaluate the accuracy of the drug-lag claims. Suffice it to say, they were and are hotly contested (Schmidt 1974; Coppinger et al. 1989). What is most important for our purposes is not the critique's validity but rather its premises and the nature of the FDA and congressional responses. For one, the critique of the FDA came in the name of cost–benefit analysis, not of consumer rights. The distinction is important. Those who objected to a reputed "drug lag" did not want to make drug law akin to securities law, where issuers can sell anything, even "bonds" they themselves claim to be "junk," so long as the prospectus properly discloses the situation. No one was urging that the consumer be left to decide among untested drugs. For another, most critics did not challenge the hierarchical control of decision making about drug therapies; they accepted the role of scientific expertise and the randomized clinical trial to evaluate efficacy. The major objection was to the use of these trials, at great expense, to ascertain the likelihood of remote side effects. Moreover, Congress generally sided with the FDA. Its main legislative response was the creation of the orphan drug program, attempting to ameliorate the problem by providing special incentives to produce drugs for small markets. Congress believed that it was not relaxing the overall standards for drug approval, but, as we shall see, the innovations in orphan drug regulation, particularly FDA participation in protocol design and expanded therapeutic use of nonapproved drugs, served as the model for changes in the AIDS era.[6]

The *fourth* characteristic of the regulatory system in the 1960s and 1970s was the adversarial posture of the regulator toward the regulated.

---

[6] 21 *U.S. Code Annotated* sect. 360bb (West Supp. 1989).

Since the drug company was "suspect," the proper stance for the FDA was to be critical and suspicious, not collaborative. It was not the role of the FDA, for example, to recommend that particular drugs be tested or to cooperate in the design of the trial. It was to be nondirective, the umpire who rules on the products developed, not a player in the game.

All of these considerations contributed to what may well be the most extraordinary fact about the drug and experimentation regulatory process: in a period when autonomy and rights were the highest values in almost every aspect of medical and health care delivery, this was one particular area in which heavy-handed paternalism flourished. Over the 1960s and 1970s, whether the context was truth-telling or the right to refuse treatment, the emphasis was on the right of the individual to make his or her own decision. Social ideology and, to an unprecedented degree, social policy reduced the discretion of those who, by virtue of their expertise, professional position, or community position, had been accustomed to making decisions on behalf of others; the list of those who suffered this loss includes college presidents and deans, high school principals and teachers, husbands and parents, prison wardens and social workers, psychiatrists, hospital superintendents, and mental hospital superintendents (Rothman 1978). But the strength of this movement notwithstanding, it was still the experts on the FDA and the IRBs, and not the patient or the subject, who decided in the first instance whether the risk/benefit ratio with a new drug or experiment was acceptable. Just when patients were securing the right to know their own diagnoses and to decide whether to accept or reject treatment, the FDA and the IRB secured the right to decide for patients and subjects whether they might try a new drug or might enter a new protocol. In essence, the arena of drugs and experimentation was an island of ideological paternalism in a sea of autonomy, running counter to the trends that swept over American medicine in the 1960s and 1970s.

The Attack on the Drug Control Model

The friction between the paternalism of the drug control model and the post-1960s commitment to individual rights smoldered rather than burned in public policy consciousness. Political life is filled with such instances, where one generation's premises lose their cultural resonance, while the bureaucratic rules and procedures they spawn continue on

nonetheless, sustained indefinitely not by the strength of their ratio-
nales but by their familiarity to the affected groups. It requires a crisis
of an unprecedented intensity to force the incongruities to a new
synthesis.

AIDS provided this very crisis. The HIV epidemic has produced a
sustained attack on the premises and structure of drug regulation and
human experimentation. Advocates for the gay community and persons
with AIDS have reacted with fury to the slow pace at which experimental therapies for the disease were sought out and initiated. As they see
it, a few cases of Legionnaires disease and a couple of poisoned Tylenol
capsules produced the scientific equivalent of a five-alarm fire. AIDS,
by contrast, claimed neither notice nor effort, and the shortfall was bit-
terly felt. Apparently, gay lives did not matter; worse yet, they might
well be intentionally sacrificed to reinforce the new conservatism's call
for a return to "traditional values and lifestyles." As a result, a coalition of AIDS advocates put forward positions that were in fundamental
opposition with those that had dominated the earlier debate (see Ap-
pendix Note). The outcome was a consumerist approach to therapy and
a powerful critique of the drug approval process. If the government
and the pharmaceutical industry were laggard in researching new therapies, then the affected community was obligated to organize itself to
track down every therapeutic possibility no matter where in the world
it might appear, and do everything that it could to make that drug
available to its members. Moreover, persons with AIDS and their advocates reject the paternalism and risk-averse attitudes of the FDA–IRB
establishment (Delaney 1989; Eigo et al. 1988). It is fascinating to recall that a mere nine years ago, the President's Commission for the Study
of Ethical Problems in Medicine and Biomedical and Behavioral Research focused public attention on the ethical dilemmas of trying out
new cancer drugs. At congressional hearings, ethicists questioned
whether researchers had not gone too far in encouraging patients' participation in "treatment" protocols for advanced cancer where there was
no likely prospect that the therapy would long delay death. To be sure,
all the patients were volunteers, but was it proper to let people in extremis volunteer for "treatment" protocols when no reasonable prospect
of cure existed? (U.S. Congress 1981). One will not see in the current
literature on AIDS any comparable concern with whether it is ethically
justified to employ experimental treatment protocols to increase, however marginally, the life expectancy of infants with AIDS.

The AIDS activists find it not only appropriate to launch initiatives to locate new drugs, but also to declare it the right of patients to have unrestricted access to these new experimental therapies (AIDS Coalition To Unleash Power [ACT UP] 1989). The fact that a therapy has not been "proved" through the canons of "good science," they assert, does not mean that access to it must be restricted, or indeed that insurers may reject claims of payment for it. Moreover, persons with AIDS reject the IRB notion that the marginal and easily exploited in our society should be protected from the risks of participation in experiments. Experimental treatment is not a burden but a form of treatment, and persons have a right to treatment, including even those who have heretofore been defined as especially vulnerable to abuse. So, for example, the American Foundation for AIDS Research (AmFAR) publishes, with government assistance, an extraordinary directory of experimental treatment to keep potential participants informed of all ongoing clinical trials. In this same spirit, activists argue that to tell a prisoner at Sing Sing that the only available medical treatment is experimental, and that he cannot for his own good participate, is to add a loss of medical benefits to the consequences of criminal conviction (Dubler and Sidel 1989).

AIDS advocates also want the FDA to be proactive, not reactive (AIDS Coalition To Unleash Power [ACT UP] 1989). In some ways, this demand requires the greatest transformation in the institutions of drug control. The structure of drug review, for the many reasons we have explored, is heavily biased in favor of caution, preserving all evaluative options until a drug company has provided fully satisfactory data. The critics, however, do not want the government to be so passive; they believe that in an epidemic it is obliged to search out any and all possible therapies, and, if necessary, to sponsor trials itself to determine a therapy's effectiveness and then publicize the results widely. The government's role should be to maximize choice, in the process providing the consumers with the information necessary to guide their decisions, not usurping their right to make decisions. In particular, the government may not use its special control over access to experimental therapies to require people to take part in placebo-controlled studies, or to limit their ability to mix and match therapies (AIDS Coalition To Unleash Power [ACT UP] 1989). The immediate interests of today's patients must come before the more-abstract and long-term interests of science and even those of future patients.

It is most intriguing that the root point of the argument, its rejection of paternalism, fits so perfectly with the pharmaceutical industry's complaints about the drug review process. For the *Wall Street Journal* and similar champions of the desire of business for deregulation, the failure of conventional medicine to offer any therapeutic hope for AIDS should be blamed on the politics and economics of the drug review process. As they see it, the AIDS shortfall is just another example of "drug lag." Rescind the Kefauver amendment requiring the FDA to measure drug efficacy, declared an editorial in the *Wall Street Journal* in July 1988, and "this single step would help AIDS patients more than any other measure currently being discussed. . . . In the midst of a medical crisis such as this, where does it say in the Hippocratic oath that patients have to accept a 1962 FDA efficacy rule . . . (based on a sedative [thalidomide] given to pregnant women) that forces half of them in these trials to accept a placebo?" (*Wall Street Journal* 1988a). The *Wall Street Journal* reiterated the theme a few months later. Taking note of AIDS advocates' recent protest against the FDA (lying on the ground outside its headquarters with hand-painted tombstones reading "I died for the Sins of the FDA," and "I got the Placebo"), the editorial, not usually supportive of such direct and theatrical street action, declared: "It has become a battle between people who have all the time in the world and people who have little time left in their lives" (*Wall Street Journal* 1989b, 1989c).

In fact, large parts of the AIDS advocates' critique of the FDA could have been scripted by the Pharmaceutical Manufacturers Association. Government must act faster, tell manufacturers precisely what it wants to know, and let consumers and their physicians decide what risks they want to run. Do not worry so much about a few injuries. Do not dally to conduct more tests on animals. When death is the alternative, get on with the job of finding good therapies. All the anger of the gay community and their ability to attract media coverage of their plight — certain to die, to die young, and with no therapies planned — serves as a lever to make palpable what is too often overlooked in the politics of drug review, namely how powerfully injured are those to whom medicine can say only, "Sorry, but we know not what to do." There is, to be sure, an incredible irony in all this. Sick gay men, abandoned by a president who refused publicly to acknowledge their disease on all but one occasion, provided the shock troops to move forward his administration's deregulatory drug control program.

While part of the AIDS critique fits perfectly well with the deregulatory plan, a large part of it does not, and the tension between the two visions is most apparent in the approaches to the randomized clinical trial. Many in the AIDS activist community reject the hegemony of scientific controls. To a much greater extent than other groups representing the victims of particular diseases, where the representation is predominantly by non-ill third parties and the group tends to become so closely allied with investigators and physicians that it functions as an interest group pressing for research funds for the medical establishment, HIV has produced critics who are not linked to medicine. For them, the system of testing should not deny individuals the right to choose their own therapeutic options simply because scientists need controls in order to determine by their own canons of evidence what works best. This is the most basic autonomy claim that consumers advance. But it leaves unanswered the critical question of how one will ever be able to know what does or does not work if there is no system to hold therapies off the market until they are tested in trials.

This then is the dilemma that has shaped the debate around drug regulation and HIV disease. Is it possible to be both proactive and protective, to facilitate medical consumerism while simultaneously guarding against the sale of snake oil, to permit people to choose for themselves while at the same time retaining the capacity to deliver, sooner or later, definitive pronouncements of what works?

The FDA's Response

Let us examine three policies—two announced by the FDA, the third a mix of FDA pronouncements and legislation—in an effort to gauge the ways in which the critique is now shaping law: first, the new rules for marketing investigational drugs; second, the thrust to make the FDA proactive; and third, the FDA's new import policy on drugs. There is an ongoing and extraordinary effort to balance conflicting demands, but whether it will be sufficient to the crisis and produce a stable and workable policy is not at all certain.

Marketing Investigational Drugs

The FDCA prohibits shipping drugs unless an NDA has been approved. The law exempts from this prohibition the shipment of drugs that are intended "solely for investigational use by experts." Complex regulations define the parameters of this exception, and detail how a sponsor gets an "IND," that is, a permit to try investigational drugs.

They also spell out the three stages: phase 1 (safety), phase 2 (efficacy), and phase 3 (clinical trials) through which new testing ordinarily proceeds (Kessler 1989).[7] In this process, sponsors have enormous responsibilities of data collection and physicians who prescribe investigational drugs are legally and contractually restricted in their use of them, bound to adhere to protocols and to report adverse effects. Ordinarily, investigational drugs are supplied free of charge to physician investigators, and through them to patients. The rationale is that these experiments are part of the sponsor's costs in proving that a drug should be allowed on the market.

In May 1987 the FDA issued rules that permit the sale of investigational drugs for serious or life-threatening diseases. Because these drugs are still undergoing testing, or data analysis concerning them remains to be done, they are, by definition, of uncertain safety and efficacy (*Federal Register* 1987).[8] To be sure, experimental drugs have been used for therapy before, particularly through so-called "compassionate use" procedures. For example, drugs to correct severe cardiac arrhythmias were made widely available through this mechanism before the FDA authorized full-scale marketing. Nevertheless, the new regime represents a formalization of authority and an encouragement to get drugs in use before their evaluation is complete.

The new regulations are complex in their attempt to balance the desirability of giving very sick patients faster access to promising therapies with the need to pursue the time-consuming and costly process of drug evaluation. To the latter end, the rules limit the investigational drugs to certain diseases, limit the distribution to certain physicians, and have a number of provisions that seek to protect the clinical trial process. They even limit the amounts that companies may charge for the investigational drugs, thereby trying to provide further incentives to complete the quest for full marketing approval. Whether these stipulations can maintain the balance between greater availability and adequate testing is far from certain. As we noted earlier, ideology and symbolism weigh heavily, and the tilt now is toward permitting patients and physicians to reach their own calculus of risks and benefits.

According to the new rules, in order to qualify for treatment status, the drug must be one that treats a "serious" or "immediately life-threatening" disease. The regulatory commentary promises a flexible approach

---

[7] 21 *Code of Federal Regulations* 312.21 (1988).
[8] 21 *Code of Federal Regulations* 312.7(d) (1988).

to defining these terms. In the regulation itself, "immediately life threatening" is defined as diseases where there is a "reasonable likelihood that death will occur within a matter of months or in which premature death is likely without early treatment" (*Federal Register* 1987).[9] The phrasing "premature death without early treatment" seems broad, and the regulatory commentary indicates that drugs that keep HIV from progressing to clinical AIDS can qualify as directed to a condition that is immediately life threatening. Inasmuch as HIV has a median latency of ten years, this seems to be a major lever by which to spread the language's reach. Moreover, the regulations do not define what constitutes a serious disease. Who will dare to label another's illness trivial? Remember the adage that minor surgery is surgery performed on someone else? It seems unlikely that any bureaucrat will relish the prospect of being called to a hostile congressional hearing to explain just why some class of sick patients is thought to suffer a disease that is not "serious." In other words, the regulations seem bounded in the class of diseases they address, but the potential for expansion, so that patients can choose faster access with higher risks no matter what the disease, is apparent.

The regulations seem to create another barrier, however. This new drug-approval route is only available to treat diseases for which no comparable or satisfactory alternative drug or other therapy exists (*Federal Register* 1987).[10] But here, too, a concept that sounds confining turns out to be much less so on closer examination. Why would a physician prescribe or a patient want to follow an experimental therapy if established treatment works? In fact, justifying experiments with new drugs when existing drugs are satisfactory is a constant issue when alternative drugs are evaluated in sick patients. The regulatory commentary makes clear that the requirement of no adequate therapy will be construed flexibly to recognize, for example, that even where approved treatments are available for a stage of a disease, not all patients respond to them. For these patients, the disease would be "serious," and inasmuch as no satisfactory treatment exists for them investigational drug use would be appropriate (*Federal Register* 1987).

The key question about the scope of the May 1987 regulations is the standard the FDA will use in deciding whether or not to permit treat-

---

[9]21 *Code of Federal Regulations* 312.34(b)(3)(ii) (1988).
[10]21 *Code of Federal Regulations* 312.34(b)(ii) (1988).

ment use of an investigational drug. The new criterion for approving this use for a drug directed to an immediately life-threatening disease is highly permissive: the commissioner must permit the drug to be marketed unless the scientific evidence, taken as a whole, fails to provide a reasonable basis for concluding that the drug "may be effective" or, alternatively, demonstrates that it would expose the patient to "unreasonable and significant additional risk of illness or injury" (*Federal Register* 1987).[11] Hence, when a drug is not particularly toxic, all that is required is some "scientific" evidence pointing toward possible efficacy. Although sheer theory will not suffice, a standard of "may be effective" precludes only those treatments for which a physician might be guilty of malpractice for recommending them. If there are some promising test results, with no sign of major toxicity, the commissioner has no legal right to restrain marketing. Whether the FDA will administer this provision so as to give full effect to its permissive language is uncertain. What is promised on paper can be modulated by administrative judgment, and it is the drug regulators who are doing the judging. Moreover, it seems highly unlikely that any large pharmaceutical company would want to litigate entitlement to a transitional designation of treatment IND. By contrast, the commissioner may deny treatment use of a drug intended to treat a "serious" disease if there is insufficient evidence of safety and effectiveness to support such use. This legal standard does not purport to control agency discretion.

If the investigational drug is approved for treatment use, it may then be prescribed by physicians who have been specially designated and recruited for this purpose. Like physicians who test new drugs generally, they must agree strictly to limit the conditions for which the drug is prescribed. Similarly, they must keep records and report adverse drug reactions to the FDA. It is not clear what other conditions may or must be imposed on the physician-selection process. While the statute assumes that only some physicians are "specially qualified" to evaluate investigational drugs, the treatment IND regulations give no hint that ordinary community physicians lack the relevant skills. Yet, the regulations contemplate using local IRBs to approve patient participation in investigational therapies. Most physicians, however, may not be associated with institutions that have IRBs. Moreover, what will it do to a

---

[11] 21 *Code of Federal Regulations* 312.42(b)(ii)(E)(1) and (2) (1988).

manufacturer's relationship with physicians if it refuses to treat them as qualified? (*Federal Register* 1987).

The manufacturer's prize under the new regulations is early access to the market and to the right to sell the drugs. To be sure, this right is not the right to commercialize the drug: it may not be advertised or promoted.[12] But again, a stipulation that seems restrictive turns out to be quite relaxed. Advertising may be insignificant if informed patient groups are prepared instantly to publicize any possible therapeutic advance and, as we shall see shortly, the government itself is pledged to keep consumers informed about potential AIDS therapies. The price that may be charged for the drug is not what the traffic will bear but rather a price limited to what will cover costs of research, production, and distribution. As a practical matter, however, the costs of research and small-scale drug production are so large that this restraint on price seems illusory. Similarly, the principle that charging for an investigational drug permits the FDA to inspect accounting records (*Federal Register* 1987) may deter some drug companies from charging.

Fears of increased product-liability exposure, and a sense of what makes for good public relations may lead firms to give away what they could sell. Most of the treatment INDs granted to date have been for products whose manufacturers have decided not to charge. For small biotechnology companies, where access to the market is everything and every nickel of product sales helps, one may find a marked reluctance to be so generous.

Perhaps a greater barrier than government limits on drug pricing will be the readiness of third-party payers to reimburse those who purchase the drug. For a number of years, the FDA's stringent requirements on proof of new drug efficacy have served as a shield by which third-party payers have resisted payment for experimental therapies. Now that the FDA is releasing drugs earlier, but without any final assertion of safety and efficacy, third-party payers face the issue of whether they should reimburse for what is still, technically, a part of the experimental process. The third-party payers obviously are on the horns of a difficult dilemma, and several so far, under pressure from advocacy groups, have agreed to reimburse before such time as the drug is finally approved. The courts may also be prepared to push them in that direction. In the

---

[12] 21 *Code of Federal Regulations* 312.7(d)(3) (1988).

recent *Weaver* decision,[13] the Eighth Circuit held that Missouri's Medicaid program could not deny funding for zidovudine (formerly azidothymidine [AZT]) although it was used for indications beyond those in the FDA-approved labeling. The Court judged that the unapproved uses were "generally accepted" by the medical community, that is, prescribed by physicians to non-Medicaid patients.

In the long run, the issue of who pays will become more and more important in the AIDS drug regulatory process, just as fiscal issues will increasingly dominate AIDS policy generally. In effect, if the government no longer bars a drug's distribution, the pressure falls squarely on the manufacturer to distribute it, and on the manufacturers and the insurers to see that those who might benefit get it. Smaller companies cannot possibly pay the full costs of a program like the one Bristol-Myers Squibb has mounted for their new drug, dideoxyinosine (ddI). The larger ones, however, may have no realistic choice, and for that reason may pressure the FDA to adopt a go-slow approach until testing is nearly complete. Similarly, the third-party payers do not want to fund pharmaceutical research and development expenses, and can also be expected to lobby the FDA to that end.

Finally, the new regulations contemplate that these investigational drug uses, with the exceptions we have noted, still must fit in under the older approval system. The new track coexists with the traditional one. Thus, the rules strongly caution that approval for this new procedure will be limited to drugs that are at the same time undergoing controlled clinical trials and whose sponsors are actively pursuing full marketing approval with due diligence (*Federal Register* 1987). It is this concern with the ongoing clinical trial process that points up the most difficult aspect of the rules. How will it be possible to maintain the clinical trial process if the drug can be obtained without the rigors of being submitted to controlled, and often placebo-controlled, trials? Where will the patients come from to join the clinical trials when the investigational drug is already available for purchase? One possible answer is from the poor, with the prospect that we will return to the days of ward medicine; in its updated version, the well-to-do will have early access to promising therapy while the poor, because they cannot afford to pay, will be left to join the clinical trials. On the other hand, con-

---

[13] *Weaver v. Reagen*, 886 F.2d 194 (8th Cir. 1989).

science may intervene in the form of an insurance provision to cover the expenses for the poor; but then the clinical trial process may well languish for want of adequate enrollments. If that occurs for an investigational treatment drug, will the FDA remove from the market a drug that clinicians report enthusiastically to be working? It seems highly improbable, even though the failure to do so will undercut the prospect of ever learning about a drug's efficacy through a randomized clinical trial.

However novel the May 1987 FDA regulations are, it should be clear, first, that they are not the lead paragraph in the obituary of the FDA. Although implementation will be affected by how the various parties respond — from pharmaceutical manufacturers to patient interest groups, from doctors to Congress and the courts — an agency that can throw a foreign nation into chaos over two tampered grapes plainly has the power to administer its rules to accomplish what it defines as necessary for public safety. The regulations are not so tightly worded as to stop them.

Second, the May 1987 rules do not explicitly incorporate a patients' rights model. Whether or not a drug gets treatment status is the decision a sponsor, almost always the manufacturer, must make. If the manufacturer chooses not to seek it, preferring, for example, not to open its books to FDA audit or to jeopardize its recruitment of subjects to a randomized clinical trial, or to render itself liable to malpractice suits because the drug turns out to be more toxic or less effective than it seemed, there is nothing that a patient seeking access to treatment can do. While a physician may seek to sponsor such treatment status, the manufacturer's readiness to go along almost always will be necessary.

Third, once the drug is on the market through the treatment exception, it is possible that the FDA will no longer feel intense pressure to approve the drug for full marketing and will, therefore, stretch out the investigational process endlessly. If that happens, the result of the regulatory innovation might well contradict the original impulse. Instead of speeding up approvals and marketing of new drugs, it will have served to increase delays.

But despite these qualifications, the potential impact of the new regulations is considerable and may well be advancing a new model of consumer rights. In particular, the standard for approving a treatment use of an investigational drug looks to patients' rights to calculate their own risks by promising access if there is evidence that a drug may be effective. It is the patient and the physician, not the FDA, that will be making a critical judgment about what drugs should or should not be taken in a war against a disease.

Toward a Proactive FDA

In October 1988 the FDA issued a second set of regulations, the so-called subpart E regulations, designed to facilitate faster evaluation of products directed to "life-threatening" and "severely debilitating" diseases. These regulations build on the ideas incorporated in the May 1987 treatment IND regulations, and commit the FDA to assisting sponsors in designing research. Subsequently, the Congress with the AIDS amendments of 1988 has committed the FDA still further to a facilitative approach to drug development. Increasingly, the government will take on the task of deciding what drugs get tested and how.

The central thrust of the October 1988 regulations is to involve the FDA in clinical trial planning, with the thought that better planning leads to shorter trials (*Federal Register* 1988). If drug sponsors are contemplating testing products that treat life-threatening illnesses or severely debilitating illnesses, the sponsor may request to meet with FDA reviewing officials early in the drug-development process to review and reach agreement on the design of necessary clinical and preclinical studies. To the extent that the products are directed to conditions with clear clinical endpoints, such as death, it should be possible to plan trials that reveal quickly whether the drug is effective. The importance of this innovation is that by involving the FDA in the very process of clinical study design, it puts an end to the adversarial posture. Studies that the FDA regards as inappropriate measures of clinical efficacy and safety will now be avoided. The potential risk of FDA involvement, however, is that by issuing a formal agreement about what must be done in order to prove a drug's worth, the FDA will find it much more difficult to rethink positions taken early on, even though it may discover important considerations that it missed earlier.

The new proposals do recognize that faster review will inevitably leave many potential problems unresolved, and, therefore, they incorporate a subtle shift in the standards for approving drugs. Thus, the 1962 statute required that drugs be proved safe and effective. But now, for products treating life-threatening or debilitating illnesses, the FDA proposes to implement this standard through a "medical risk-benefit" approach. In effect, the FDA will permit the marketing of drugs whose safety parameters are still unknown, if the benefits look substantial. It will then seek to ascertain the answers about the precise range of treatment effects and dangers while the drug is on the market. Yet, unlike the situation with the 1987 treatment INDs, where only physicians who agree to act as investigators and live by the reporting rules may have access to the drug, under these new regulations the drug is actually on the market. Any physician is free to use it for whatever purpose, subject only to the discipline of potential malpractice liability and perhaps the refusal of third-party payers to reimburse nonindicated uses. Again, the central issue is the feasibility of a two-track system, continuing closely controlled investigations while permitting general use.

Two other aspects of the October 1988 regulations warrant brief mention. First, the FDA proposes to make its 1987 treatment provisions applicable to drugs that are fast-tracked in this manner. Thus, a drug might be made available for sale if promising data appear in early phase 2 studies, so that data from perhaps as few as 200 patients will suffice to get a drug on the market and earn its sponsor money. Second, the FDA has indicated in these regulations that it is itself prepared to carry out some of the critical testing as part of a regulatory research program. For example, the FDA may do the work to develop assays or determine necessary manufacturing standards. Here, too, the changes promise to reduce the expenses of drug innovation.

These rules are potentially of enormous benefit to the United States biotechnology industry, long filled with promise but short on products. To a greater extent than conventional pharmaceuticals, the new biotechnology products are based on an understanding of disease processes at the molecular level and in genetically engineering products to respond. Successes are more likely, if they come at all, to be demonstrable with small sample sizes. The new rules have the potential to reduce dramatically the costs of reaching the market by, in effect, eliminating the entire process of phase 3 clinical trials, the most expensive part of the clinical testing process. By getting money back faster, small biotechnology companies have a greater chance of holding on to their own products, rather than having to license them to more established companies.

Congress appears fully supportive of the innovations we have outlined. Indeed, in the AIDS amendments of 1988, it went beyond the FDA in the extent to which it gave legislative support to a consumer-rights approach to drug development. The 1988 law requires the establishment of an AIDS Clinical Research Review Committee within the National Institute of Allergy and Infectious Diseases.[14] The committee must be composed of physicians whose clinical practice includes a "significant number" of AIDS patients. It has affirmative obligations to advise on research on drugs that might prove effective in treating HIV. The committee is to recommend to the secretary of the Department of Health and Human Services new drugs for which preliminary evidence indicates effectiveness in treatment or prevention of HIV, and the secretary is to publish that fact in the *Federal Register* and encourage an application for investigational use. Having done so, the law also directs the secretary to encourage the sponsor to seek a treatment IND so that the drug will be available, and if the sponsor does not do it, it authorizes the secretary to encourage physicians to become sponsors of treatment INDs on their own.[15] Perhaps even more important, the law mandates the creation of a data bank on controlled clinical trials which persons with AIDS can have access to, and it even obliges the government to test whatever underground drugs the community, in fact, is using.[16] Thus, the initiation and control of drug testing is moving from the experts to the community, and the community is to be kept constantly apprised of each nuance of development—the better to be able to secure access to therapy without undergoing placebo-controlled trials.

The Import Policy

The greatest concession to consumer entitlement is the recently announced policy of the FDA permitting importation of drugs for personal use. Unlike the other policies we have considered, this one is not embodied in statute or regulatory language but results from a proclamation of the commissioner concerning the ways in which the enforcement authority of the FDA would be exercised in the future (U.S. Department of Health and Human Services 1988). In essence, the FDA has announced that anyone can have access to any drug in the world so long as a physician agrees to supervise its use.

As the recent experience with Chilean grapes makes clear, the FDA

---

[14]42 *U.S. Code Annotated* sect. 300cc-3 (West Supp. 1989).
[15]42 *U.S. Code Annotated* sect. 300cc-12 (West Supp. 1989).
[16]42 *U.S. Code Annotated* sect. 300cc-16 (West Supp. 1989).

has broad authority to exclude from the United States products that do not comply with United States requirements. In the past, the FDA had exercised that authority vigorously to keep out, among other things, laetrile, when groups had organized to procure it in Mexico and distribute it to cancer victims in the United States. The power to exclude an unproven drug intended for the terminally ill was confirmed by the Supreme Court in *United States v. Rutherford* in 1979.[17]

Nonetheless, at a 1988 National Lesbian and Gay Health Conference and AIDS Forum, the commissioner of the FDA presented a new policy on imports of drugs. Any person, not only those with AIDS, may import drugs if the product is intended for personal use; if the product is not for commercial distribution and the amount of the product is not excessive (a three-month supply); and if the intended use of the product is appropriately identified and the patient seeking to import the product provides the name and address of a supervising licensed United States physician. If these conditions are met, the individual may not only bring the drugs across the border himself, but may use the mails as well.

The policy represents a striking departure from the FDA's prior insistence on its legal duty to enforce the prohibitions on introducing unproven drugs into United States commerce. Still, it is easy enough to understand the extraordinary pressure the FDA was under. Unlike the cancer situation, where there are many plausible treatments for most cancer patients, there are only a handful of approved treatments to recommend for AIDS. Moreover, as a practical matter, the nation cannot police its borders to prevent determined AIDS activists from simply traveling abroad and returning with drugs whose shipment is permitted in foreign countries but forbidden here. (The failure to keep out heroin and cocaine is surely a lesson in point.) Although the announced policy amounts to a surrender by the FDA of its role as protector of consumer health by certification of drug safety, at least it has the virtue of requiring some physician involvement, and it provides a basis for policing to some extent the worst kinds of health fraud. Thus, when a Canadian company announced its intention to lower its price of dextran sulfate and facilitate mail orders to the United States, the FDA moved immediately to block it on the grounds that the company's activities amounted to improper commercial promotion (Boffey 1989).

While the FDA's approach may represent a pragmatic accommoda-

---

[17]442 U.S. 544 (1979).

tion, the symbolic implications of the move are striking. People are permitted to shop for therapy worldwide, and make their own determinations about whether the risks of treatment are outweighed by potential benefits. The elaborate procedures of American law for protecting against inappropriate risk taking, including IRBs and informed consent requirements, are entirely lacking. To be sure, if a foreign drug looks like it is killing people, the word will get around soon enough, and the government will no doubt be active in spreading the word. But this is government as editor of *Consumer Reports*, not as the protector of sick people from exploitation. Moreover, the import policy is not restricted to AIDS but applies to any medical consumer, at least to anyone who has the resources to go abroad in order to receive treatment there first.

In the long run, easy toleration of imports may play havoc with other aspects of the United States pharmaceutical industry. One of the consequences of the FDA's change in policies, and faster grants of permission to market drugs, is that third-party payers will be increasingly restive at paying for expensive treatments simply because the FDA has allowed them on the market, without a finding of safety and efficacy. These new therapies will often be very expensive, especially those that have been produced by the new genetic engineering technologies. Will the economic returns that the developers of these therapies hoped for be undercut by imports of similar drugs produced abroad at lesser prices? Finally, progress in treating AIDS is likely to come incrementally and, like cancer treatments, be built on careful combinations of drug regimens to produce maximum destruction of infected cells with as little damage to healthy ones as possible. For these purposes especially, although the point is generally true about clinical trials, it is important to limit the compounds the experimental subject is taking. If experimental subjects have access to a wide variety of alternative therapies, and use them either to augment the effect or protect against the failure of the medications they are receiving in controlled trials, then the sample sizes of clinical tests will have to get bigger in order to account for the variability that these unauthorized remedies induce. This will undercut, however, the entire thrust of the movement to run smaller but better-designed trials to get the drugs on the market faster. In this same fashion, to the extent that new drugs appear on some foreign markets faster than they do in the United States, the availability of compounds abroad constantly undercuts the incentives to participate in placebo-controlled clinical trials.

Parallel Tracking

The pressure on federal bodies to speed up the distribution of investigational drugs is so intense that proposals are now being offered and endorsed without prior attention to substance or procedure. The most vivid example of this process at work is the "parallel track." First suggested in July 1989 by the director of the National Institute of Allergy and Infectious Diseases, and quickly backed by the director of the FDA, the purported purpose is to make available to patients drugs that have moved through phase 1 tests and are about to enter phase 2, that is, drugs that have been demonstrated safe with some prospect of efficacy. The initial proposal, however, made no mention of the treatment IND program, obfuscating the question of how, if at all, the two programs differed.

Between July 1989 and May 1990, government and advocacy groups worked to give explicit content to the parallel track program. The issues ranged from the kinds of data that merit enrolling the drug in a parallel track to the types of patients who should be eligible to receive the drug and the appropriate evaluative data as well. Understandably, different groups had different agendas. Some saw the parallel track as an opportunity to run larger trials, and thus to secure more data. Others wanted to divorce entirely the parallel track from all research efforts. But the underlying problem remained: how did the parallel track expand access beyond that permitted by the treatment IND? After all, where drugs are directed at life-threatening diseases, the treatment IND regulations go very far toward permitting the marketing of promising drugs. The drug has only to meet a "may help and no proof of harm" standard. What room is left, then, for further expansion of access through the parallel track? Is it proposed to move the point of widespread use back even earlier and make drugs available where it cannot plausibly be said that "the scientific evidence taken as a whole" supports the judgment that the drug *may* help?

On May 21, 1990, in a notice of proposed policy, the Public Health Service (PHS) issued the first regulatory embodiment of the parallel track concept. It is not accidental that the proposals were issued by the PHS and not the FDA, which had been acceding to demands for consumer choice, for the policy represents a retreat from the ideology of the treatment IND and the liberalized drug import policy.

The proposed policy would permit individuals with AIDS and HIV-related diseases to take promising investigational agents. The only patients who are eligible, however, are those who are not able to take standard therapy, those for whom standard therapy is no longer effective, and those unable to participate in the relevant clinical trials. Here the parallel track proposal is actually more restrictive than the treatment IND regulation. In those regulations, it was not patient characteristics but patient–physician preference that determined whether the drug released on treatment IND would be obtained. The sponsoring company had a general obligation to move ahead with full-scale evaluative procedures, including trials, but if those clinical trials were ongoing, any patient, not just those who had failed at other therapy, could, with the physician's approval, take the new drugs. The parallel track proposal, by contrast, narrows the patient pool. Trials come first, and patient choice is subject to their imperatives.

The proposed policy undercuts the permissive language of the treatment IND in yet another way. The new policy states only that a treatment IND "may" be granted—not "shall" be granted, as per the original language—after sufficient data have been collected to demonstrate that the drug "may be effective" and does not carry unreasonable risks. It makes the treatment IND discretionary rather than mandatory when the evidence suggests that the drug may be effective. In effect, in order to make room for a parallel track, the prior standard is ignored— although, to be fair, the FDA itself had been taking a narrow view of the regulation's power. Nevertheless, inasmuch as the treatment IND only requires evidence that the drug "may" be effective, it is difficult to imagine a standard lower than this as consistent with believing that one has any scientific evidence whatsoever.

Conclusion

What, then, should we expect of drug regulation in the future? Clearly, the FDA has been engaged in an exquisite balancing act, attempting to respond to the AIDS-related criticisms without abandoning what it considers to be fundamental principles of good medical science. Can this balance hold? The history that we have been tracing suggests that the tilt is, and will be, to a consumer-rights orientation. Perhaps the events of the past two years represent a strategic retreat on the part of the FDA that will ward off a more total defeat, but it is highly unlikely that the FDA will soon again enjoy the authority that it possessed in the 1960s and 1970s.

There is good reason to anticipate that we will witness increased innovation and less concern for risks in drug development and human experimentation. The nightmare cases have changed; thalidomide and Willowbrook are no longer the ruling images. The number of new drugs for AIDS coming onto the market will increase, and if many turn out to be ineffective, some may accomplish a degree of good. The losses will be forgotten in light of the victories, even if they are slim.

Events that transform policy in the realm of AIDS will not be limited to AIDS. As consumer-rights notions advance in this one disease, they will be (indeed they are already) picked up by other similarly situated groups and their advocates, whether afflicted by Alzheimer's disease or Parkinson's disease. If these groups were originally too "doctor-oriented" to lead the change, they are not so "doctor-oriented" to stand out against the change. Indeed, the FDA in both its May 1987 regulations and its 1988 importation policy is framing its response to look beyond AIDS to other diseases. Hence, we have every reason to expect that the ranks of advocates for opening up procedures will be expanding, coming to include not only those who have long wanted to see deregulation affect federal policy (Reagan's supporters and proponents of a drug-lag thesis) but a variety of patient groups who find themselves victims of disease with no readily effective treatment. In essence, the consumer movement will be contagious, making it all the more likely to spread and to be successful.

The lock of the university investigator on clinical trials will not be maintained. The incentives to other physicians to enter into the process will be high, and they will inevitably come from a variety of backgrounds and be affiliated with a variety of types of institutions. The tertiary medical center locus for trials will weaken and along with it the singular dominance of the randomized clinical trial as necessary and sufficient "proof."

However staunch the FDA defense of its prerogatives, the concessions that it has already made — and will have to continue to make — will mean that consumers and their doctors will be forced to make difficult decisions without substantial information at hand. There is bound to be more guess work, more hunches, more variety, ultimately more "schools" of medicine — reminiscent of but never quite duplicating the array of schools that characterized American medicine in the nineteenth century. It will be less feasible to define orthodoxy, more impossible for the patient — and for the physician as well — to cite unimpeachable authority. It will be much easier to establish patient self-help groups. *Consumer Reports* is likely to have many analogues in medicine.

Biotechnology firms will flourish, able to reach markets more quickly and, therefore, able to command capital more easily. They will have to withstand the pressures from imported drugs, but they may well be able to compete more effectively with them. Indeed, we might even witness a proliferation of drug researchers, and some successes with a few patients may well be a road to incorporation and financial windfalls. To be sure, the incentives to fraud will increase (if it only takes a sample of 100 patients to get access to the market, how tempting it will be to manipulate the recruitment of subjects and resulting data) and, all the while, knowing what is or is not fraudulent will be that much more difficult.

How far the example set in drugs will spread to other products is not easy to estimate, but it would not be astonishing were product-liability laws weakened (with the drug case raised as the precedent). Let the buyer beware may well be the credo of the future.

Medical insurance companies and other third-party payers will face the most acute dilemmas in deciding what therapies deserve reimbursement. They will have strong incentives to become more conservative — not underwriting every drug that hits the market, especially in light of how costly the drugs will be. But their reluctance will generate counter pressures, and even regulation compelling them to underwrite "unproven" therapies. The rates they charge are bound to increase, thereby giving more fuel to the fire of a national health insurance scheme. Of course, national health insurance costs would also mount, but not so precipitously as to make it seem absurd to spread the cost of insurance more broadly through some type of national system.

Finally, and with near certainty, the pendulum will swing again: The accumulation of failures will slowly affect public policy. Another thalidomide or Willowbrook scandal will eventually resume its hold on the public imagination, and the FDA will assume more of its older authority. Protection will gain in favor, the enthusiasm for innovation at all costs will wane, and the cycle will begin all over again.

Appendix Note

We are well aware that the constituent groups that advocate on behalf of persons with AIDS are diverse and often disagree on policy questions. The AIDS "community," like other communities, can and does divide on a variety of issues, including the ones we are analyzing here. (The propriety of running underground and unofficial drug trials is a case in point.) But our goal here is to analyze the general consensus that unites most advocates and hence our use, relatively undifferentiated, of the term "advocates for persons with AIDS," and "AIDS advocates and activists."

References

AIDS Coalition To Unleash Power (ACT UP). 1989. *A National AIDS Treatment Research Agenda.* Issued by ACT UP and distributed at the Fifth International Conference on AIDS, Montreal, June 4–9.

American Foundation for AIDS Research (AmFAR). 1990. *AIDS/HIV Experimental Directory* Vol. 4, No. 2 (June). New York: AMFAR.

Beecher, H.E. 1966. Ethics and Clinical Research. *New England Journal of Medicine* 274:1354–60.

Boffey, P.M. 1988. U.S. Bans an AIDS Drug from Canada. *New York Times,* August 2.

Congressional Record. 1962a. Drug Industry Act of 1962. 17395–405.

——. 1962b. Drug Amendments of 1962. 22315–25.

Coppinger, P.L., C.C. Peck, and R.J. Temple. 1989. Understanding Comparisons of Drug Introductions between the United States and the United Kingdom. *Clinical Pharmacology and Therapeutics* 46(2):139–45.

Delaney, M. 1989. The Case for Patient Access to Experimental Therapy. *Journal of Infectious Diseases* 159:416–19.

Dubler, N.N., and V.W. Sidel. 1989. On Research on HIV Infection and AIDS in Correctional Institutions. *Milbank Quarterly* 67(2):171–207.

Eigo, J., M. Harrington, I. Long, M. McCarthy, S. Spinella, and R. Sugden. 1988. *FDA Action Handbook.* Washington: Federal Drug Administration. (Mimeo., September 21.)

Faden, R.R., and T.L. Beauchamp. 1986. *A History and Theory of Informed Consent.* New York: Oxford University Press.

Federal Register. 1971. Institutional Committee Review of Clinical Investigations of New Drugs in Human Beings. 36:5037–40.

——. 1987. Investigational New Drug, Antibiotic, and Biological Drug Product Regulations: Treatment Use and Sale. 52:19467–77.

——. 1988. Investigational New Drug, Antibiotic, and Biological Drug Product Regulations. Procedures for Drugs Intended to Treat Life-Threatening and Severely Debilitating Illnesses. 53:41516–24.

Frankel, M.S. 1973. *The Public Health Service Guidelines Governing Research Involving Human Subjects.* Monograph no. 10. Program in Policy Studies in Science and Technology. Washington: George Washington University.

Inside R&D. 1990. New Drug Development Costly. May 2.

Kaitin, K., N. Mattison, F.K. Northington, and L. Lasagna. 1989. The Drug Lag: An Update of New Drug Introductions in the United States and the United Kingdom, 1977 through 1987. *Clinical Pharmacology and Therapeutics* 46(2):121–38.

Kessler, D. 1989. The Regulation of Investigational Drugs. *New England Journal of Medicine* 320:281–88.

Klerman, G.L. 1974. Psychotropic Drugs as Therapeutic Agents. *Hastings Center Studies* 2:81, 91–92.

Lasagna, L. 1989. Congress, the FDA, and New Drug Development: Before and After 1962. *Perspectives in Biology and Medicine* 32:322–43.

Rothman, D.J. 1978. The State as Parent. In *Doing Good*, ed. W. Gaylin, S. Marcus, D. Rothman, and I. Glasser. New York: Pantheon.

———. 1987. Ethics and Human Experimentation: Henry Beecher Revisited. *New England Journal of Medicine* 317:1195–99.

Newsweek. 1989. August 7.

Schifran, L.G., and J.R. Payan. 1977. The Drug Lag: An International Review of the Literature. *International Journal of Health Sciences* 7:359–81.

Schmidt, A.M. 1974. *Testimony before the Subcommittee on Health of the Committee on Labor and Public Welfare, and the Subcommittee on Administrative Practices and Procedure of the Committee on the Judiciary, U.S. Senate.* Examination of the Pharmaceutical Industry 1973–74, August 16, 2949–3139. Washington.

Sherman, J. 1966. Letter to Roman Pucinski, July 1. National Institutes of Health files, Washington. (Unpublished.)

Trials of War Criminals before the Nuremberg Military Tribunals. 1949. Washington.

U.S. Congress. 1981. *National Cancer Institute's Therapy Program: Joint Hearings before the Subcommittee on Health and the Environment of the Committee on Energy and Commerce (House of Representatives) and the Subcommittee on Investigations and Oversight of the Committee on Science and Technology (Senate), 97th Congress, first session,* October 27, Washington.

U.S. Department of Health and Human Services. 1988. FDA Talk Papers, July 22 and 27. Pilot Guidance for Release of Mail Importations. *Food and Drug Law Reporter,* Commerce Clearing House, para. 40,923.

Wall Street Journal. 1988a. AIDS and 1962. July 14.

———. 1988b. The FDA for Itself. October 13.

———. 1988c. New Ideas for New Drugs. December 28.

Wardell, W. 1973. Introduction of New Therapeutic Drugs in the United States and Great Britain: An International Comparison. *Journal of Clinical Pharmacology and Therapeutics* 14:773–90.

Acknowledgments: This project was supported by a grant from the American Foundation for AIDS Research, and their assistance is gratefully acknowledged. We also benefited from the counsel and research of Hazel Sandomire, associate research scholar at the Julius Silver Center for Law, Science, and Technology, and Joel Zinberg, May Rudin Fellow at the Center for the Study of Society and Medicine.

Part III.

Systems of Caring

The Culture of Caring
AIDS and the Nursing Profession

RENÉE C. FOX, LINDA H. AIKEN, and
CARLA M. MESSIKOMER

Caring is nursing and nursing is caring (Leininger 1984, 83).

Nurses provide care for people in the midst of health, pain, loss, fear, disfigurement, death, grieving, challenge, growth, birth, and transition on an intimate front-line basis. Expert nurses call this *the privileged place of nursing* [emphasis added] (Benner and Wrubel 1989, xi).

Nursing has always been a much conflicted metaphor in our culture, reflecting all the ambivalence we give to the meaning of womanhood. Perhaps in the future it can give this metaphor, and ultimately caring, new value in all our lives (Reverby 1987, 207).

THE NURSES WHO SPEAK THROUGH THESE quotations all agree that caring is, and always has been, the cornerstone and the quintessence of their profession. It is the key concept of nursing, the vital theme around which the whole field turns. Coded into the notion of caring are the characteristic forms of knowledge and skill, practice, and ritual, the fundamental attitudes and values, beliefs and symbols that define the work that nurses do, its goals, its meaning, and its distinctive culture.

Over time, the world in which nurses work has undergone fundamental alterations that have diminished the paramountcy of caring, making it more difficult to sustain on a consistent and continuing basis. Changes in illness patterns, the increasing dominance of technology in medical care, the growth of bureaucratic medicine, and the preoccupation with cost containment in recent years all act to constrain and thwart nurses from meeting what they regard as their foremost and unique obligation to patients. This commitment is succinctly expressed in the motto on the 1989 American Nurses' Association National Nurses' Day poster: "Our Caring Is Constant." In the face of the many circumstances that deter nurses from acting upon their underlying belief that "[c]aring is nursing and nursing is caring" (Leininger 1984, 83), it is remarkable that caring actually occurs so much of the time.

The amount of attention that the American nursing profession has paid to the principles and the phenomena of caring has increased steadily during the 1970s and 1980s. This is especially apparent in the subject matter and discourse of articles, textbooks, monographs, and dissertations that nurse-scholars trained in anthropology, psychology, sociology, education, history, and philosophy have been writing and publishing, and in the statements of educational philosophy and objectives that have been issued by schools of nursing in recent years (Watson 1979, 1985; Benner 1984; Tisdale 1986; Wolf 1988). The current reemphasis on the supremacy of caring in nursing and on its association with the very identity and raison d'être of the field emanate from important ideological, intellectual, and clinical developments that are occurring within the profession.

Against this background, we will examine the nursing profession's "culture of caring" in detail — its contents, sources, modes of transmission, and the ways that it is brought to bear on the AIDS epidemic. We shall then consider some of the consequences that nurses' involvement in taking care of persons with AIDS may have on the conditions and environment of their professional work, on their collective outlook and morale, and on their relation to the larger health care system.

Since 1965 the trend in nursing education away from diploma schools and toward colleges or universities has greatly accelerated. In 1965, 80 percent of new nurse graduates were trained in hospital diploma programs; by 1986 fewer than 15 percent of new graduates were from hospital programs while more than 80 percent graduated from two- and four-year college programs (Aiken and Mullinix 1987). In addition, the contemporary women's movement has had a significant effect on the outlook of the overwhelmingly female membership of the nursing profession (96 percent of registered nurses). The presence in the profession of a critical mass of highly and broadly educated nurses, and of women with raised feminist consciousness, has contributed to a surge of activity directed toward more systematically and fully conceptualizing, describing, and studying the caring core of nursing as, for example, in this excerpt from the writings of nurse-anthropologist Madeleine Leininger (1980, 135, 141–42):

> Caring behaviors, processes, and structures are the most central and unifying focus of nursing practice, and should comprise the major intellectual, theoretical, practical and research endeavors of nurses. . . . Care [should be] studied in a systematic way: a way which explores linguistic usage, epistemologic sources and cross-cultural examples of care and their relationship to nursing. . . . The resulting scientific and humanistic body of nursing knowledge should improve client services by developing an in-depth perspective on the very core of nursing. . . . It will help to validate and explain the distinct nature of nursing.

The preoccupation of the nursing community with the importance of "uncovering" and authenticating what is "embedded" (Benner 1984, 3-4) in their own precepts and practices of care has been accompanied by a drive to distinguish their field from the profession of medicine by which it has been historically dominated, and to liberate nursing from some of the fettering aspects of its inherited definition as "women's work." As will be seen, this has entailed an intricate process of trying to attain some distance from what historian Susan M. Reverby (1987, 1 and in passim) terms the "ordered to care" tradition of nursing, while asserting its "right" and "desire" to care. It has also involved concerted efforts to demonstrate rigorously that caring attitudes and behaviors such as touching, feeling, and comforting, which are culturally regarded as "feminine" and "soft," are not only "virtuous," but have positive clinical effects on patients' health, illness, and disease that are scientifically explicable.

The same period of renewed interest in caring in nursing has also been a time of crisis for the profession, marked by a serious shortage of nurses, growing discontent among nurses with hospital employment, high rates of "burnout" and job turnover, and a dramatic decline in nursing school enrollments, and in the number of persons planning to pursue nursing careers (Aiken and Mullinix 1987). The enhanced interest in caring is, in part, related to this crisis, which has been increasingly linked to nurses' perceived loss of control over their practice—particularly over their ability to care for patients in a manner consistent with their deeply held values (Maslach and Jackson 1982; Kramer and Schmalenberg 1988; Kramer and Hafner 1989). It is at this complex juncture in the evolution of the American nursing profession that the interrelated epidemics of human immunodeficiency virus (HIV) infection and acquired immunodeficiency syndrome (AIDS) have appeared on the national scene.

AIDS is unique among diseases in present-day societies because it is simultaneously acute, chronic, progressive, infectious, and fatal—and also affects young people. At our present stage of medical knowledge, there is no cure for the total collapse of the body's immune defenses that the AIDS virus causes. Despite recent improvements in pharmacologic therapies, for the great majority of symptoms that plague people with AIDS—ranging from the irritating to the excruciating—there are simply no substitutes for the hands-on, face-to-face forms of physical and interpersonal care that constitute the very core of nursing, and in which nurses, above all other health professionals, excel.

Key Components in Nursing Care and Its Culture

> Caring for the sick is a queer way to spend one's time, and we act as though it were the most normal thing in the world (Tisdale 1986, 5).

The most basic and palpable aspects of the work that nurses do pertain to the bodies of the patients for whom they care. Nurses attach great significance to caring through touch—even in highly technical health care situations where they refer to these caring actions as "high touch" (Brody 1988, 93).

As Zane Robinson Wolf (1988, 180–230) has shown, bathing patients is one of the most important physical and symbolic foci of these corporeal dimensions of nursing. It is a practice that not only "belongs to the domain and responsibility of nursing," but also contains within it some of the distinctive attributes of the bodily care that nurses render. The explicit scientific rationale for the bath is "to protect the patient's skin, the first line of defense against disease." It entails handling "private bodily parts," and "dirty," potentially dangerous and contaminating "infected materials, excreta, such as urine, perspiration, and stool, and secretions, such as mucus, blood, and wound drainage." As nurses recognize, bathing patients is more than an epidermal and hygienic set of procedures. It is also a highly structured, expressive enactment of some of the cardinal values and meanings of nursing care. Skill and grace, comfort and healing, intimate nonverbal as well as verbal communication with patients, respect for their dignity and privacy, and rituals of order, protection, and purification are all combined in the optimally conducted bed bath.

Both in principle and in fact, nursing care is a continuum. It entails an ongoing relationship to patients in all phases of illness and of the life cycle, including dying and death; and it calls for what philosopher Milton Mayeroff (1971, 34, 43) terms "the constancy . . . [of] being with the other." These continuity dimensions of nursing care are epitomized and also sanctified by the "last office"-like procedures that nurses perform when a patient death occurs. ("Even after patients die," Zane Wolf [1988, 139] writes, "nurses care for them, touching them with gentleness.") Bathing the dead patient, laying out his/her body for viewing by the family, and for transport to the morgue, and cleaning the patient's room are constituent elements in what is known as "post-mortem care" in the language of nursing:

> The symbolic meaning of the post-mortem ritual rests in the nurses' need to remove the manifestations of suffering, to purify the patient's body and hospital room of the soil and profanity of death, and to gradually relinquish their tenure of responsibility for the patient, given up only as the escort personnel transport the patient to the morgue (Wolf 1988, 139).

In death, as in life, great importance is attached to the role and the meaning of the laying on of hands. To be sure, in their delivery of modern scientific care, nurses do not use only themselves as therapeutic instruments; they bring complex machines and other forms of high technology to bear upon the caring process. They value these advanced modes of care, and have professional pride in their competence to utilize them. But, nurses recognize that absorption in technological medicine can drive a wedge between them and their patients, "dehumanizing" the care that they give, and they worry vociferously about this:

CCU [Critical Care Unit] nurses ran in and out of the room, bringing in supplies as they were needed. Lori, the supervising nurse,
stood in the corner with pen and paper, recording every action,
while Luce, with her back to the rest of the room, concentrated on
the monitor, calling out the rhythms as they came over the screen.
    No one was looking at Mrs. Nelson, the scared, dying woman.
    The resuscitation stopped as a normal heart pattern smoothly slid
across the monitor screen, and Mrs. Nelson again began to breathe
spontaneously.
    A desire to comfort her engulfed me, and I gently pushed my way
to her side. Recognizing me, she started to cry and grasped my hand
(Heron 1988, 300).

In common with most of her colleagues, Echo Heron, the critical-care
nurse who wrote this, also experienced "a great feeling of satisfaction"
when she "removed all the tubes and wires" from a patient's body, in
the first phases of post-mortem care — "as if I were purifying him"
(Heron 1988, 239) — and she valued "peaceful deaths . . . unimpeded
by the resuscitation technology of the defibrillator, monitor, ventilator,
and electrocardiograph" (Wolf 1988, 139).
    These sentiments are associated with the perspective on the human
body that is inherent to nursing. It is a more holistic conception than
the one that underlies the biomedical model. In this nursing view, the
body is not an object that is separate from, or external to, the thoughts
and feelings, the experiences and relationships, the life history and the
"self" of the individuals for whom nurses care as patients. Rather, "the
influence between mind and body is [seen as] synergistic and mutual,"
and "the body [as] continuous with the person." In turn, this notion of
the body has "profound implications" for the way that nurses approach
and care for their patients' bodies, especially for the "messages of comfort and activity" that they believe they can, and should transmit to patients in this way (Benner and Wrubel 1989, xii, 53).
    The nursing outlook not only includes recognizing and responding
to the entwined physical, emotional, and social aspects of health, illness,
and caring, but also encompasses what nurses refer to as their "spiritual"
dimensions. These are the human-condition encounters with new and
old life, suffering and tragedy, mortality and death, and with the questions of meaning they elicit that nurses intimately face with patients
and their families.
    Ideally, a caring relationship with patients as defined by nursing en-
tails a dynamic "turning toward the other" meeting of nurse and pa-

tient, through which the nurse enters and empathically shares the patient's situation and suffering. By being present with patients in this compassionate sense, and using herself, as well as her knowledge and skill, therapeutically, the nurse provides comfort and support to them and to their families; relieves their physical, emotional, and existential distress; promotes their developmental growth and change (and her own as well); and creates a climate in which healing, if not always cure, takes place. "Perceptual awareness" and "discretionary judgment," devotion, trust and hope, courage, respect, and something akin to love for the person who is one's patient are all constituent elements of this ideal model of nursing care and caring (Gaut 1979, 23–24).

Caring about, for, and with patients in these ways includes serving as "health educators" for them and their families — sharing information with them, and teaching them skills that are pertinent to their illness situation and conducive to their well-being. In addition, nurses are expected, and taught, to translate their caring commitment to patients into "patient advocacy" when it is called for:

> The nursing ethos of the past, rooted in unquestioning obedience to the physician, has given way to an ethic of advocacy for the patient. The present American Nurses' Association [1985] Code for Nurses, for example, dictates that respect for human dignity and support of the patient's rights to self-determination are an integral part of nursing practice. Furthermore, when patients lack the capacity to decide, nurses are expected to act in their best interests, operating from a patient-oriented rather than a medically-oriented perspective (Theis 1986, 1223).

Nurses' Socialization for Caring

The science and philosophy of nursing care — its concepts and principles, knowledge and skills, and the attitudes, values, and beliefs that underlie it — are central to the process of professional education. In part, nursing care is taught to them through lectures, in the classrooms, laboratories, and clinics of their nurses' training, and via the textbooks, articles, and manuals that they study en route. The manner in which nurses learn the methods and ethos of caring that are distinctive to their profession, however, is not confined to these forms of pedagogy. In fact, it might be said that it is largely through other media that the culture of caring is conveyed to nurses.

Preeminent among these is the way in which nurses are socialized to acknowledge the feelings that their lived-in experiences with patients arouse in them, and to share these experiences and feelings with each other. Coping with the stresses of caring in this fashion is a preferred means of coming to terms with difficult emotional, moral, and spiritual aspects of their work, which nurses are explicitly encouraged, and taught to use:

> Health care workers are repeatedly exposed to breakdown, tragedy, and death. Even with the best defenses, the nurse must confront the limits of control, and inevitability of death, and in the case of violence, the very real presence of cruelty. Nurses know through their work that the worst can happen, and this infiltrates and colors one's sense of the world. Health care workers may cope with laughter, bravado, detachment, and elaborate self-protective maneuvers to feel immune to the calamity they confront, but these are temporary "Band-Aids" that can grant only fleeting immunity. In the midst of such "immunity-granting" coping, it is helpful to acknowledge to one's coworkers the pain and threat one confronts (Benner and Wrubel 1989, 376-77).

The nursing profession imparts its cultural tradition of caring to neophytes most powerfully through its participatory mode of teaching them the procedures that constitute the major "occupational rituals" (Bosk 1980) of their field. These are highly patterned, finely regulated practices that are "part of the fabric of the personal-care tasks" (Wolf 1988, x) that nurses perform in their daily rounds. On an unspoken and symbolic level, they contain within them key values and goals that are integral to the identity of nursing and the meaning of nursing care. Zane Robinson Wolf's study of nursing rituals on "7H," a medical unit in an urban teaching hospital, singles out post-mortem care, medication administration, medical aseptic practices, and change-of-shift report as among the most important of these at-once "sacred and profane" aspects of nurses' work (Wolf 1988).

As Wolf observed, despite the existence and easy availability of hospital policy and procedure manuals that detail these practices, they are not generally used in training nurses. Rather, the procedures are taught chiefly by demonstration, and by oral transmission in everyday practice as well as demonstration contexts. Some of the more symbolic and sacred aspects of these nursing care acts are nonverbally communicated: for example, "the tradition of not crossing the arms of a Jewish patient" (Wolf 1988, 121) in giving post-mortem care. The fact that these ritual-infused acts of nursing are conveyed from one generation to another in a practicum setting, through face-to-face interaction, oral tradition, and structured silence, enhances their conscious and unconscious impact on both senior and junior nurses.

Social Origins of Nurses and Their Ethos of Care

While we acknowledge the deep influence that their education and clinical experiences have on nurses' socialization in caring, we believe that the social origins of nurses also play a significant shaping role in this process.

The best time-series data available on the social backgrounds of nurses, and some of the attitudes and values relevant to care and caring with which they begin their professional education, are found in the annual survey of entering freshmen in American two- and four-year colleges and universities that has been conducted since 1966 by the American Council of Education–University of California, Los Angeles (ACE–UCLA) Cooperative Institutional Research Program (CIRP). These 23 years of data about college freshmen include within them a population described as "aspiring nurses," (i.e., students planning to major in nursing) who are overwhelmingly female in gender. Compared with the women "nonnurses" (i.e., those planning careers other than nursing), in the 1988 CIRP freshmen survey, these nurse aspirants have the following sociodemographic characteristics and value orientations that we feel are relevant to their entry into the profession (Astin, Green, and Korn 1987; Green 1987; unpublished data from the Higher Education Research Institute of the University of California, Los Angeles 1989).

The standard indicators of socioeconomic status—parental income and education—suggest that a sizeable proportion of nurse aspirants are products of working- and lower-middle-class families. Prospective nurses are much more likely to come from lower-income families than freshman women interested in other careers: one-third of the nurses compared with only one-fifth of their nonnursing peers reported a parental income under $25,000 per year. An examination of the sources of funding for educational expenses on which nurses rely is further suggestive of the economic status of their parents. Compared with other freshman women, nurses are more likely to have received federal grants and loans based on economic need to finance their education; a significantly smaller proportion have received contributions in excess of $1,500 per year from their parents for college expenses (43.7 percent versus 64.2 percent), and more than twice as many nurses as nonnurses expect to work full time while attending college.

Nurse aspirants also have a lower proportion of parents who are college educated than the nonnursing population: less than one-third of "nursing fathers" compared with more than one-half of the fathers of their nonnursing contemporaries were college graduates. The same pattern holds when mothers' education is considered. The educational status of "nursing parents" is even more starkly revealed by the 1986 CIRP survey data, which showed that their percentage was the lowest among all "professional parents," including parents of aspirants to allied health fields and to elementary and secondary school teaching.

The data on fathers' occupations, for the most part, do not provide meaningful comparisons since many of the occupations listed are imprecisely defined. (For example, the category of "businessman," into which a substantial percentage of both "nursing and nonnursing fathers" fall, does not differentiate among managerial, sales, and support positions within the private sector.) By collapsing the lower tiers of the occupational ladder, however, where definitional clarity prevailed, some sense of the differences between the two groups emerges. One-quarter of "nursing fathers" held jobs classified in the survey as skilled, semiskilled, or unskilled, or were unemployed, versus 14.8 percent of the fathers of their nonnursing peers.

Finally, with respect to their religious orientations, nurse aspirants were preponderantly Christian. Of these, the largest proportion was Catholic (36.9 percent), while Baptist was the next most frequently cited denomination (20.7 percent). More than twice as many nonnurses as nurses reported no religious affiliation.

The same freshman survey has identified a number of attitudinal and value patterns that distinguish nurse aspirants from their nonnurse peers and appear to have some bearing on their prospective entry into nursing:

- Nursing students gave greater support to the life goals of "helping others in difficulty" (83.2 percent versus 66.3 percent) and to "raising a family" (76.8 percent versus 67.5 percent).

- They were somewhat less likely to endorse "being very well off financially" as an "essential" or "very important" life goal, although they more frequently cited "getting a better job" or "making more money" as a rationale for pursuing a college education.

- The nurse aspirants were somewhat more inclined to have attended religious services during the year prior to the survey, while laying less emphasis on "developing a philosophy of life" than the nonnurse population. While fewer nurses rated this item as an "essential" life goal, their embeddedness in the ethos, if not the institution of their religion, may have already provided the philosophical underpinnings that more of their college peers cite as a "very important" life objective.

The extent to which nursing students' social class, religious origins, and value orientations influence their socialization to the culture of caring in nursing is an issue that has rarely been raised, and the answer remains elusive. The virtual and puzzling absence of discussion on this topic by both nurse-scholars and sociologists who observe, study, and inform the profession about its values and attitudes, beliefs, and practices—both latent and manifest—represents a significant void in the literature on the socialization of nurses. The cognitive, technical, and attitudinal aspects of being a nurse are communicated, explicitly and implicitly, through an intensive, highly structured process. But students do not arrive in professional school as empty vessels, devoid of values, attitudes, and beliefs. Nurses carry into their professional education the constellations of values that their family, social class, and religious origins have helped to shape. The role that these background factors play in the professional socialization process, and the degree of their complementarity to the core value of caring in the nursing profession merits further investigation. Whatever the extent of their impact, we would expect that a change in the social origins of prospective entrants to the profession would alter, in critical and observable ways, the culture of caring.

In addition, these same factors may also help to account for the unusual allegiance that nursing students have to their chosen field. Even as freshmen, they appear to have developed clearly defined career choices to which they are strongly committed. A comparison of responses of nurse and nonnurse aspirants to a number of questions concerning their "probable" college major and future career plans reveals striking differences. While fewer than 4.5 percent of the student nurses expect to change their major or their ultimate career goal, this was the case for 18.2 percent of the nonnursing freshman respondents. And, given the significant attention which the current and anticipated nursing shortage has received in both the manpower literature and the mass media, it is not surprising that 90 percent of the nurse aspirants expect to find employment in their field of choice. Although these data reflect expected rather than observed changes in career preparation and occupational preference, they are, nonetheless, suggestive of the unusual degree of attachment these nurse aspirants have, so early in their education, to the profession of nursing and the culture of caring in which it is grounded.

Nursing Care of Persons with AIDS

> Because AIDS is a chronic life-threatening illness that has no cure, it is essentially a nursing disease—that is, the essence is caring rather than curing (Fahrner 1988, 115).

Caring for persons with AIDS calls upon the entire range of physical, psychological, social, and spiritual interventions that nurses are characteristically, and, in many respects, singularly educated to provide. It encompasses home and hospice care delivered in the community, as well as acute-care nursing in the hospital. And its most technically proficient and humane forms are predicated on the "compassionate holistic" (Fahrner 1988, 121) conception of care around which nursing's professional culture turns.

The chief physical symptoms and sources of suffering with which AIDS nursing care is concerned, and that nurses attempt to manage and relieve, include pain which is often severe; disabling fatigue and weakness; grave nutritional problems; chronic diarrhea, which leads to numerous secondary problems, including skin breakdown; sensory and perceptual deficits related to neurological involvement; anxiety, depression, and dementia; fevers; and the ever-present threat of infection (San Francisco General Hospital Nursing Staff 1986; Memorial Sloan-Kettering Cancer Center; California Nurses' Association 1987; Durham and Cohen 1987; *Journal of Palliative Care* 1988; Lewis 1988; World Health Organization in collaboration with the International Council of Nurses 1988). To this appalling syndrome of simultaneous, multiple disease processes that are severe, progressive, and affect virtually every organ system of the body, and to the serious side effects that are engendered by some of the medications used to treat the symptoms of AIDS (particularly opportunistic infections), nurses bring every caregiving skill that they "always use with patients." "Nursing care of acutely ill patients with AIDS does not require a new body of knowledge," they assert (Fahrner 1988, 115). In the sphere of physical care, the nurse must marshal sophisticated observational and assessment skills to identify and evaluate signs of impaired gas exchange and neurological alterations contributing to the patient's respiratory and sensory-perceptual difficulties. This care also relies on such use of practical, time-honored comfort and security measures, as giving patients chicken broth to counteract the metallic taste induced by pentamidine, a drug used to treat pneumocystic carinii pneumonia (PCP); turning and positioning patients and massaging their bony prominences frequently while they are in bed, keeping their sheets wrinkle-free, and lubricating their skin with a mixture of vitamin A and D ointment and mineral oil to prevent skin breakdown; encouraging patients with painful lesions of the oral mucous membrane to take cool, soothing nourishments (i.e., ices, jello, ice cream, malts); and providing patients with calendars, clocks, photographs, familiar objects, signs identifying their room and bathroom, and the like, as ways of contravening central nervous system disease-induced mental confusion, and minimizing the necessity for using restraints. In addition, the AIDS nursing care plans and published descriptions of nursing interventions recommend the employment of "innovative, creative" methods (Fahrner 1988, 118)— notably, alternative pain control therapies (therapeutic touch, relaxation exercises, guided imagery, and visualization), and "holistic approaches to spiritual, emotional, mental and physical well-being to enhance general immune response" (Nurses' Coalition on AIDS as published in California Nurses' Association 1987).

Caring for persons ill with AIDS elicits all of nursing's psychological, social, cultural, and educational expertise, and its spiritual care-giving capacities as well. The young, mortally ill AIDS patients to whom nurses continually minister and relate are not only riddled with many forms of physical suffering. They are also beset by a communicable,

epidemic disease that is greatly feared in the general population, and
even among many physicians, nurses, and other health care professionals. It is also a disease that (at the present time in the United States)
primarily afflicts "many people whose lifestyles are different from the
majority of the society," as the Memorial Sloan-Kettering Cancer Center nursing care plan for AIDS euphemistically puts it. The fact that a
large proportion of people with AIDS are homosexual or bisexual men
and intravenous (IV) drug users has evoked widespread stigmatizing,
shunning, and discriminatory reactions to persons with AIDS, along
with the more fearful ones that expose them to isolation and rejection
and make them more vulnerable to feelings of shame and guilt. Furthermore, the diagnosis of AIDS can force persons ill with it to reveal
their homosexuality or their drug abuse to family, loved ones, friends,
and colleagues who may respond with anger, anxiety, fear, or revul-
sion. In addition, the disease ravages the bodies of those who have
AIDS in ways that may drastically affect their self-image and repel
others. The extreme weight loss that accompanies AIDS, and the thick,
purplish tumors of Kaposi's sarcoma that develop under the skin are
among the most publicly visible and disfiguring signs of the disease.
And hovering over it all is the fatality of AIDS: the imminent, youth-
fully premature death that so far has claimed every person afflicted with
the disease.

> I . . . wish to thank the nurses on 10 East, whose genuine concern
> and lack of fear made Peter's six hospital visits at UCSD Medical
> Center bearable. Their excellent care helped us and continues to
> help so many others. . . . I have an ever-growing admiration for his
> nurses. Peter is but one of many AIDS patients with [the] problem
> [of diarrhea with incontinence], but they go about their chores very
> matter-of-factly and treat him with respect and affection. They come
> and go constantly, asking how he feels and encouraging him to talk
> about his feelings. He seems to feel their concern for them, too.
> When he was admitted yesterday, he went first to the nursing sta-
> tion. . . . He feels very comfortable in their care (Peabody 1986, ac-
> knowledgments, 135).

This tribute, written by a mother whose son died from AIDS at the
age of 29, testifies to the crucial role that nurses and the care that they
render play in helping persons with AIDS, their families, and significant others to deal with their psychic, social, and spiritual suffering:

with the fear and anxiety, anger and angst, the isolation and ostracism, guilt and shame, the change in self-image, the loss of self-competence and self-worth, the sense of helplessness, and of putrefying decay, the sorrow and despair, and the ultimate questions of meaning that the AIDS situation engenders in them. Particularly during the multiple in-hospital stays that AIDS patients undergo, it is the nurses who are not only the most continuous, immediate, 24-hour providers of care in all these spheres, but also the chief coordinators of the kind of holistic, multidisciplinary, collaborative caring that is involved. This nursing-integrated model of care is centered on the patient, in relation to his/her family and significant others. In addition to nurses and medical doctors, it draws into its orbit psychiatrists, social workers, nutritionists, respiratory and physical therapists, clergy, and community-based AIDS services, among others. Along with pain and symptom management, nursing care plans for AIDS emphasize understanding illness from the viewpoint of what persons afflicted with the disease, their relatives, and intimates experience, and also from inside the emotions that it arouses in nurse caretakers. It is a model that includes persons with AIDS in decision making and self-care as much as possible, while enabling them to accept the assistance they need; educating and counseling patients and those close to them about matters vital to coping with the illness and with impending death; and creating conditions that can foster "peace of mind and spirit," through the existential growth both of the persons suffering from AIDS and of those caring for them. These conceptions and dimensions of care, and the values they embody are the foci of the various nursing care plans for AIDS that we have examined. Written in the disciplined and systematic language of the scientific method, these plans are nonetheless full of highly practical and deeply humane prescriptions for nursing care and caring (Becknell and Smith (1975).

Social Contexts of AIDS Nursing

Nurses care for patients with AIDS in a number of different settings, both inside and outside the hospital. The various organizational contexts in which they work, and the roles that they assume in these milieux, are as expressive of their caring philosophy and convictions as the specific nursing acts that they perform.

Inside the hospital, acute AIDS nursing care is carried out within relatively small, "designated" or "dedicated" units, as they are known, which are exclusively for AIDS patients, or on regular, inpatient services, where "scattered beds" of persons ill with AIDS are located. Some 40 American hospitals now operate special AIDS units, representing 750 beds in 10 states and Puerto Rico, and the number of such facilities is steadily increasing (Taravella 1989). A model for many of them is the pioneering Special Care Unit of San Francisco General Hospital, opened in July 1983, which was planned by the Hospital's Department of Nursing (Morrison 1987). Some of the social systems, as well as nursing and medical attributes of oncology, burn, and clinical research units have also influenced the conception of specialized AIDS care units. The two types of arrangements for hospitalizing AIDS patients reflect a growing debate regarding the best strategy for organizing AIDS care.

Proponents of dedicated AIDS units point to the overall advantages of specialized units, including staff who are experienced and expert in managing the type and range of problems presented by AIDS patients, and who are able to provide continuity of care over time. Furthermore, staff on special AIDS units become particularly knowledgeable about how the disease is transmitted. As a result, they may more accurately assess and more selectively use isolation precautions, thus giving less expensive and more humane care. The specialized units appear to be more conducive than general hospital units to developing the whole spectrum of required services, integrating inpatient and outpatient care, and involving an interdisciplinary team. In addition, patients may feel less stigmatized and more open in a specialized unit where everyone shares common difficulties and hopes. In specialized units, patients often have roommates who are companions in suffering and sources of support, whereas in other units AIDS patients are often isolated in private rooms. From an educational perspective, specialized units offer nurses, physicians, and other health professionals the opportunity to rotate through the AIDS service and to concentrate on the challenges of HIV infection without the distractions of competing clinical priorities.

The opponents of the concept of specialized units argue (without any confirmation at this time) that the nursing staff will "burn out" more quickly if they are exclusively devoted to the care of AIDS patients, and that the units will pose difficult recruitment problems.

There is also some fear that hospitals with dedicated units will become known as "AIDS hospitals" which will scare away other patients. The possibility that special units may end up isolating and stigmatizing people with AIDS in ways analogous to the situation of patients in mental hospitals has been raised, along with the speculative prediction that, in the long run, this could lead to a deterioration in the quality of AIDS care. Finally, the practical matter of costs has been invoked; unless a hospital can expect a stable and high census of AIDS patients, it is alleged, a dedicated unit with its fixed costs can be considerably more expensive than admitting AIDS patients to whatever hospital bed is available.

Definitive institutional answers to these questions have not yet been reached. But from the perspective of our interest in nursing's culture of caring, it is significant to note that many of the nurses affiliated with AIDS units have volunteered to work in those settings, and that a number of these units have sizable waiting lists of nurses eager to join them. For these nurses, it would seem, some of the most important values, meanings, and fulfillments of their profession are epitomized in this sort of intensive, expert, primary nursing-centered team environment, where the mission is to care skillfully and compassionately for the very ill persons whose fatal conditions cannot be cured in a supportive, holistic, and collaborative patient-and-family-oriented way that involves both the individuals who suffer from AIDS and their caretakers in a therapeutic community. We have seen no evidence to substantiate the thesis that nurses who elect to work in special AIDS units are different from other nurses, either demographically or in their sexual orientation. Instead, we are inclined to believe that nurses tend to be attracted to AIDS and other specialized units primarily because the degree of professional autonomy and support that they are accorded in these settings help them to provide what they regard as quality care.

The activities of nurses involved in AIDS care are not confined to the hospital, but extend beyond it into the homes of persons with AIDS, where public health nurses, visiting nurses, home care nurses, and hospice nurses, among others, play a central role in assessing, monitoring, managing, and treating the "roller-coaster nature of the disease" at all points "along the continuum of [the] illness, from the time an individual is at risk for infection through [its] terminal phase" (Dickinson, Clark, and Swafford 1988, 216).

From the earliest days of the epidemic, nurses have assumed strong roles in developing such volunteer- and community-based AIDS services, and as care providers within them. For example, "the first meeting of the KS [Kaposi's sarcoma] Foundation, which later evolved into the San Francisco AIDS Foundation, was held in a school gymnasium, and was organized and led by health care providers, including a nurse, a hospital administrator, and a physician, working with two or three community organizers" (Lewis 1988, 307). Nurses have continued to be active in this foundation, which offers community and professional education and counseling services relevant to AIDS, support groups for persons with AIDS, their families, and significant others, and transportation facilities.

Nurses have also been pivotally involved in the Gay Men's Health Crisis, Inc. (GMHC) since this premier AIDS voluntary association in New York City was founded in 1982. As GMHC has grown in volunteer membership and staff, and expanded its educational, hot-line, counseling, support group, home care, case management, crisis intervention, transport, and research activities, nurses — themselves volunteers — have helped to structure, coordinate, and administer these functions. Their input has been especially important in GMHC's "buddies" program. This consists of some 700 to 1,000 volunteers, organized in teams of from 9 to 15 individuals, who help persons with AIDS living at home to manage the daily rounds, by assisting them with housekeeping tasks, grocery shopping, meal preparation, laundry, personal grooming, and the like; by keeping watch over their medical condition; and by providing them with a supportive, caring presence. Each "buddy team" functions under the continual aegis of a nurse, a "captain," and sometimes a "co-captain"; and it meets once a month as a group. Nurses in GMHC not only engage in supervisory and organizational functions; they also do a certain amount of hands-on care as "buddies," case manager partners, and crisis interveners (J.A. Bennett, personal communication 1989).

Anecdotal evidence suggests that a considerable number of nurses are volunteering their free time to care for people with AIDS in home and hospice settings. As Rashidah Hassan (executive director of Blacks Educating Blacks about Sexual Health Issues) explains, "Nurses are drawn to volunteering [because it] allows for personal expression. They're not locked into a system," the way nurses are when they carry out their daily hospital-based work round. As volunteers, nurses "can do hands-on, direct education and . . . physical caring and comfort on their own terms" (American Nurses' Association 1988, 23). Above and beyond the gratifying autonomy that nurses experience in volunteering, we find it an impressive confirmation of their commitment to caring that so many nurses have the motivation and the stamina to extend their care giving into their after-work, personal lives.

The several organizations we have mentioned are examples of what has been estimated to be the over 500 agencies related to AIDS that have developed in the United States since the recognition of the epidemic (Lewis 1988). Chiefly in and through such organizations, and both the national and state levels of the American Nurses' Association, nurses have also been involved in policy and political advocacy activities to ensure that financial and community resources are made available to provide skilled, humane care for all persons with AIDS, and to promote continuing public and professional education relevant to the prevention and treatment of the disease.

Challenges and Stresses of AIDS Care Nursing

This is not to say that American nurses are massively participating in caring for AIDS patients, or in AIDS-associated activities. Nor do we mean to imply that—impelled by their profession's moral commitment to deliver care without prejudice to all those who need it, regardless of the nature of their health problem, social or economic status, or personal attributes—all, or even most nurses are unambivalently ready to respond to the suffering and danger that AIDS has brought in its wake. Various surveys of nurses' attitudes toward AIDS and caring for patients with the disease that have been conducted in different regions of the country indicate that, in common with many physicians and other health care professionals and workers, a sizable number of nurses feel great reluctance about caring for AIDS patients, because of their fear of infecting themselves or family members, their disapproval of homosexuality and discomfort about relating to homosexual men, their strong negative sentiments about intravenous drug use and users, and because of the relentlessly fatal outcome of the disease (Douglas, Kalman, and Kalman 1985; Blumenfield et al. 1987; Wertz et al. 1987; Colombotos 1988; van Servellen, Lewis and Leake 1988a, 1988b).

Even those nurses highly committed to caring for persons with

AIDS, and experienced in doing so, admit that there are aspects of taking care of AIDS patients that they find "devastating." Most frequently
mentioned in this connection is the lethalness of the disease:

> DONNA GALLAGHER: . . . There's futility in this disease. We
> have never been faced — at least not in my lifetime — with the kind
> of epidemic where everyone experiencing it is probably going to die.
> People die of cancer but you have a phase where you can really
> cheerlead them on and hope that they get by. With AIDS, there's
> really not a cheerleading phase.
>   We all feel the pressure that no matter what you do, or how hard
> you do it, or how fast, you probably won't save anyone. That's a
> very big obstacle that we have to get by as nurses.
>   JOAN L. JACOB: When someone asks me, "What's the hardest
> thing for you?" I say, "Grieving. There's not enough time."
>   I lost 125 patients in about a year and a half. When I am review-
> ing charts, maybe 50 at a time, I say to myself, "They are all dead."
> Then it hits me and I begin to grieve anew for each one. . . .
>   We are not prepared for this. But how can you prepare people for
> something this devastating? (Bennett 1987, 1150–55).

Nurses also experience stressful difficulties in caring for AIDS patients who are IV drug users; these are not as likely to be mitigated
over time as the anxieties that many of them initially bring to the care
of AIDS patients who are homosexual. In contrast to the gay persons ill
with AIDS who are predominantly white, with above-average educational and income levels, drug users with AIDS in cities like New York
are mainly Hispanic or black, with no more than a high school education or less, whose incomes have often been reduced to poverty through
the psychic and social, as well as the financial, costs of getting and taking drugs. While AIDS is increasingly becoming a disease affecting
blacks and Hispanics, the racial and ethnic composition of the nursing
profession remains overwhelmingly white. In 1988, 91.7 percent of the
over two million licensed registered nurses in the United States were
non-Hispanic whites (unpublished data from the National Sample Survey of Nurses, U.S. Department of Health and Human Services 1984,
1988). In this respect nurses and the patients with AIDS for whom
they are caring are culturally dissimilar. Nurses have not written about
these sociocultural differences between themselves and their patients.
They do report difficulties, however, in establishing good nurse/patient

relations with IV drug users who have carried into the hospital context distrusting attitudes and manipulative behaviors characteristic of street drug culture (Friedman et al. 1987).

The Redeeming Significance of Caring for Persons with AIDS

Written in the tradition and rhetoric of personal witnessing, testimonials composed by nurses have appeared both in the nursing literature and in the print media. They express a quickened, reconverted, and recommitted relation to the primary values and ultimate meaning of nursing and nursing care. AIDS and nursing those afflicted with it are not only portrayed in their particularities; they are also viewed as "writ large," collective representations of disease and illness in general, and of the "legacy" of "car[ing] for others the way we would want to be cared for if we were sick." Beyond that, they are linked to societal issues of justice and equality, and of individual rights and communal responsibility, and to transsocietal, universalistic principles of dignity, love, peace, and panhuman oneness.

I have just spent 12 hours in a darkened room with a man who exudes fury and despair. Disagreeable, rude, scathingly critical, he lies wrapped in blankets because he is always cold, an angular bony heap, too weak to hold a newspaper without effort, too dejected even to try, shut down from whatever life he has left. Refusing to complain, he hugs his misery to himself like a cloak of thorns.

He has AIDS. . . .

Ordinarily, I scoff at knee-jerk responses to AIDS, those panicky overreactions vastly disproportionate to the facts. But after my first night of caring for someone with AIDS, I plunge straight into paranoia, tumult, confusion.

The barrage is a shock. I went into this nursing with open eyes. . . . I know how [AIDS] is transferred and how it is said not to be transferred. I understand that people who suffer from this terrible illness have a damn good reason to be angry, frightened, depressed. I even took a course that taught me how to deal with all of this. But, in fact, I am not prepared. . . .

As I sit at my desk, I think about the man to whom I am scheduled to return tonight. . . . Does it occur to him that I have come to

him out of choice? In my imagination, I say to him, "I am here because I believe that every human being has a birthright to stand
whole and proud of who he is and, in times of trouble, to be cared
for with love and respect." . . .

I climb into bed with a cup of hot milk. I am calmer, more reflective. But the negative feelings aren't so easily banished, nor should
they be. . . . I remind myself that wearing gloves does not have to
be inharmonious with concern, compassion, courtesy. . . . Further,
my responsibility is to seek guidance and support for myself so that
I can continue to do this work and do it well (Worth 1988, 60, 62).

. . . I entered Michael's room and introduced myself. I stretched
out my hand – as I had done in many other rooms – but Michael
turned away and kept his hands hidden beneath the bedcovers. "I
have AIDS," he said rather tersely. "You've got to wear a space suit
to come into this room. Didn't they tell you?" "I'd like to shake
your hand and talk to you awhile," I offered. "I'm not afraid. Are
you?" Michael turned toward me in disbelief. Slowly he pulled
away. Tears appeared and rolled gently down his thin face. "This is
the first time my skin has touched the skin of another person for 12
days," he wept. . . .

During one year with Michael, we formed the AIDS Nursing Task
Force, an *ad hoc* group in which we shared knowledge about AIDS.
The "space suits" disappeared from our wards, and with the confi-
dence and courage we now felt, . . . we were able to share our new
insights with parents, physicians, dieticians, and housekeepers. . . .

Michael is gone, but he left a powerful legacy: through him, we
have been able to see the simple truth of caring – to care for others
the way we would want to be cared for if we were sick (Brock 1988,
46–47).

Although the language of such testimonials is not explicitly religious, either in referring to a deity or in a denominational sense, they
are infused with the Christian ideas of *caritas*. (The historical fact that
nursing originated in Christian religious orders, and the contemporane-
ous fact that the majority of present-day American nurses are Christian,
among whom many are actively identified with their religious tradition, probably contribute to the importance of *caritas* in the caring
ethos of the profession.) Another notable feature of these testimonials
is the degree to which they turn around an in-depth encounter with a
particular patient, who has become for the nurse/witness, and in many
cases for her/his colleagues, too, the personification of the moral and
spiritual, as well as medical import of AIDS.

Reflections on the Long-term Effects of the AIDS Epidemic on Nursing

What kinds of enduring effects, if any, will the advent of AIDS in its epidemic form, and nurses' response to it, have on the profession's view of itself; on the way that it is regarded by others (physicians and other health professionals, patients and their families, and the public at large); on the social system of the hospital in which nurses are the chief and most constant providers of around-the-clock care; and on the multiple extrahospital and community settings where nurses do their work as well? Deciding how to address these questions—what to look for and look at—is an intricate matter; venturing predictions of this sort is highly speculative at best. Experts of various kinds who have attempted to forecast what the long-term impact of AIDS on nursing will be have expressed divergent opinions. On the one hand, for example, in stating their concern about the availability of an adequate number of nurses to care for AIDS patients, the Presidential Commission on the Human Immunodeficiency Virus Epidemic (1988, 23) commented:

> The acuity of disease of persons with HIV infection, the complexity of their physical and psychosocial needs, the high fatality rate, and the fear of exposure to HIV, along with low salaries and understaffing in many facilities, create a potential for considerable stress, burnout, turnover, and dramatic projected shortages for the delivery of HIV patient care in the near future. On the other hand, as we have seen, many of the nurses who have spearheaded the profession's involvement in AIDS care are convinced (to quote one of them) that "it has taken the AIDS epidemic for us to develop a vision for the future and realize our true potential as a profession": AIDS offers us many opportunities for growth. . . . Working with AIDS, as with other illnesses, can be extremely trying and stressful. Although it constantly tests our abilities as professionals and individuals, it does not have to be depressing. We can find unlimited fulfillment in our work with these patients, their families, and their significant others and walk away knowing we have done our best. AIDS continues to test our society; those of us who accept the challenges and face the issues head on will find a personal fulfillment and satisfaction that we have never known before (Morrison 1988, xviii-xvix).

Our perspective on the ramifying consequences that AIDS will have for the nursing profession is both more tentative and more complex than either of these extreme positions.

It appears to us that a critical mass of the nurses working in the field of AIDS are, indeed, having an extraordinary opportunity to use their profession's "particular ability to care" (Witcher 1987). What is more, they are exercising it in a way that bridges what historian Susan Reverby describes as "the dichotomy between the duty and desire to care for others and the right to control and define this activity" with which nurses — and others who do what our society considers "women's work" — have long contended (Reverby 1987,1). Since there is presently no cure for AIDS in sight, it is only caring, and caring of precisely the sort that nurses are uniquely trained to perform, that makes a difference. As a result, in most AIDS care settings, nurses are not only the chief dispensers of care; they also play central roles in directing and coordinating it. Furthermore, nurses are gaining recognition from physicians, as well as from patients and their families, for their caring attitudes and competence. This is especially true in the designated AIDS units that hospitals have created:

> The nurses on the AIDS unit [at Montefiore Medical Center in New York City] say their job satisfaction is related to being treated more respectfully than usual by physicians. . . .
> Dr. [Gerald] Friedland [medical director of the unit] agreed that AIDS has altered the traditional relationship between doctors and nurses. Nurses, he said, adapted more easily to situations where patients were comforted rather than cured.
> "They were trained that way and we weren't," Dr. Friedland said. "My generation of doctors were all of the belief we could cure everything. We have become more modest" (Gross 1988).

In these respects, it would seem, at least in AIDS contexts, that the role of caring, and the distinctive relation of nursing to it have been receiving significant interprofessional and institutional acknowledgment. What is more, the kind of care that is being responded to in these ways exemplifies the knowledge and skills, attitudes and values that the leading "philosophy and science of caring" spokespersons of the nursing profession espouse, and are trying to convey to the new generation of students entering the field. The AIDS situation has even helped to loosen the tight association of nursing care with "women's work," through the conspicuous number of male nurses who are engaged in the clinical care of AIDS patients.

Particularly in some of the cities where the AIDS epidemic has reached crisis proportions, it has been a catalyst for organizational change and innovation in the delivery of AIDS care. For example, the San Francisco General Hospital has developed what is nationally considered to be a model system of comprehensive, multidisciplinary, physical, and psychosocial care of patients with AIDS, that emphasizes out-patient management, and integrates it with inpatient services and also home care—working in close collaboration with a network of community agencies to achieve this (Volberding 1985). Nurses, both male and female, have been instrumental in designing this system, and in implementing it through the plethora of care-giving and care-administering roles they fill within it. Many of the organizational features that characterize these new AIDS service programs incorporate elements long sought by nurses, and have been recommended by the series of expert panels on nursing that were convened during the 1980s (Institute of Medicine 1983; National Commission on Nursing 1983; U.S. Department of Health and Human Services 1988), but which have rarely been put into practice by health care institutions. The dedicated AIDS units are among the most noteworthy of these.

But will these changes that, at one and the same time, improve care for persons with AIDS and the working situation of nurses, persist in the settings where they are already in place? Will they spread to other facilities and communities? And will these AIDS-induced patterns and models of care influence other parts of the health care system through a sort of spillover effect? For a variety of reasons, our prognosis is guarded.

To begin with, some of the factors that have been essential to the favorable developments that have occurred in AIDS care and nursing only exist in certain locales. One such precondition has been the presence in particular areas of many gay persons who "have built a wide range of political, social, and community organizations," which have "served as an infrastructure" for their collective response to AIDS (Friedman et al. 1987, 202). Within this framework, in cities like San Francisco and New York, they have played a crucial part in creating an ensemble of community-based services for AIDS patients, and in linking them with both the inpatient and outpatient care provided by hospitals.

The priming role of the gay world in fostering new forms of AIDS care is relevant to another phenomenon that could eventually undermine what has been achieved. Up until now, gay males have been the main risk group for AIDS in cities such as New York and San Francisco; but the number of new HIV infections among gay males has significantly declined. The number and proportion of intravenous drug users with AIDS, however, has been increasing. As we have indicated, the majority of drug users with AIDS are poor, black, or Hispanic, with low educational levels, whose ability to organize themselves to deal with AIDS is seriously hindered by "individual, subcultural, and societal obstacles" (Friedman et al. 1987, 215). Will the care organizations that have developed in response to AIDS be willing and able to absorb this influx of disadvantaged and disenfranchised persons into their midst? And if so, will this bring about other creative changes in the system of AIDS care; or will the challenging demands involved progressively lead to its erosion and deconstruction?

In the long run, in particular cities where the growth in AIDS patients continues, more of whom are poor and underprivileged than in the past, this may plunge the already overburdened health care system of the community into a grave state of crisis. Such is currently the case in New York, as a mayoral panel of health experts appointed to examine the AIDS situation in the city reported in March 1989:

> There are 1,800 AIDS patients in hospitals in New York City. Most hospitals are reporting that they are filled to nearly 100 percent capacity. . . .
> Acquired immune deficiency syndrome "is tearing at the very heart of the city," the report said.
> "AIDS is not only the city's medical crisis of our times," the panel added, "but threatens to become the city's social catastrophe of the century.
> "AIDS did not create the crisis, but it now represents the final straw, which threatens the well-being of the entire system and the availability of health care for all New Yorkers."
> Without remedial action, the panel warned, "the whole proud New York City system of patient care, biomedical research and medical training, generally viewed as the best in the world, will swiftly deteriorate" (Lambert 1989).

In appraising the possible long-term effects of the AIDS situation on care and caring, nurses and nursing, and on the relations between them, what also needs to be considered as a limiting factor is the relative "invisibility" of the new models of care, and of the singular role of nurses outside the AIDS-circumscribed universe. For all of their real advantages, for example, this may turn out to be one of the major drawbacks of designated inpatient AIDS units. Their relative insularity within the hospital, along with their specificity, may make them too inconspicuous to affect the hospital as a social system.

What is more, many nurses who are engaged in AIDS care feel that what they are doing and what they know are not being adequately seen or heard, either inside or outside the hospital:

> DONNA GALLAGHER: One obstacle is that nurses in this field are invisible. You hear physicians being interviewed about the crisis and even about patient care issues. But do reporters interview nurses?
>
> JOAN L. JACOB: Unfortunately, [nurse] clinicians are so busy that they don't have time to go out and be heard. Our energies at the end of the day are in going home and healing our wounds.
>
> GAYLING GEE: For such a high-profile disease, nursing certainly has kept a very low profile. As much as we do, we need to talk about it more (Bennett 1987, 1151–52).

Nurses are perhaps most conscious of still another factor likely to constrain the long-lasting influence that AIDS can be expected to have on the health care system, and on the recognized place of nurses within it. This is what might be called an historical forgetting process. Most people are unaware that many of the challenges and issues that AIDS presents are not unique, first-time occurrences. This nonawareness carries with it a lack of acknowledgment of the important care initiatives that the nursing profession has taken in the past:

> PAT McCARTHY: Everything is so reminiscent of what happened in oncology 20 to 30 years ago. AIDS is a new disease but it has raised the same old issues. When there were no specific community resources for people with cancer, nurses had to insist that existing community resources be used to treat people with cancer or to offer their home care services to people with cancer. Well, now we're telling the community agencies, "You may not realize it, but all your services are going to apply to people with AIDS, too." We're in the position of convincing people that they need to take on one more disease category (Bennett 1987, 1152).

When that day arrives to which we all look forward, and AIDS has become a disease that is more within our power to control, will the part that nurses have played at this juncture in its history be recalled? And whenever it is that we reach the point of being able to cure, as well as prevent, AIDS, will we continue to appreciate the lessons about the importance of caring that it has taught us, and of the embodiment of the skills, the values, and commitments that it entails in the work and the culture of the nursing profession?

We hope so. And we hope, too, that what we have written here will contribute to the remembering.

References

Aiken, L.H., and C.F. Mullinix. 1987. The Nurse Shortage: Myth or Reality? *New England Journal of Medicine* 317:641–46.

American Nurses' Association. 1985. *American Nurses' Association Code for Nurses, With Interpretive Statements.* Kansas City.

American Nurses' Association. 1988. *Professional Heroism, Professional Activism: Nursing and the Battle against AIDS.* Kansas City.

Astin, A.W., K.C. Green, and W.S. Korn. 1987. *The American Freshman: Twenty Year Trends, 1966–1985.* Los Angeles: Higher Education Research Institute.

Becknell, E.P., and D.M. Smith. 1975. *System of Nursing Practice: A Clinical Nursing Assessment Tool.* Philadelphia: F.A. Davis.

Benner, P. 1984. *From Novice to Expert: Excellence and Power in Clinical Nursing Practice.* Reading, Mass.: Addison-Wesley.

Benner, P., and J. Wrubel. 1989. *The Primacy of Caring: Stress and Coping in Health and Illness.* Reading, Mass.: Addison-Wesley.

Bennett, J.A. 1987. Nurses Talk about the Challenge of AIDS. *American Journal of Nursing* 87:1150–57.

Blumenfield, M., P.J. Smith, J. Milazzo. S. Seropian, and G.P. Wormser. 1987. Survey of Attitudes of Nurses Working with AIDS Patients. *General Hospital Psychiatry* 9:58–63.

Bosk, C.L. 1980. Occupational Rituals in Patient Management. *New England Journal of Medicine* 303:71–76.

Brock, R. 1988. Beyond Fear: The Next Step in Nursing the Person with AIDS. *Nursing Management* 19:46–47.

Brody, J.K. 1988. Virtue Ethics, Caring, and Nursing. *Scholarly Inquiry for Nursing Practice* 2:87–96.

California Nurses' Association. 1987. *AIDS Resource Manual.* San Francisco.

Colombotos, J. 1988. The Effects of Caring for AIDS Patients on Attendings, House-Staff, and Nurses. New York: Columbia University School of Public Health, Division of Sociomedical Sciences. (Unpublished.)

Dickinson, D., C.M.F. Clark, and M.J.G. Swafford. 1988. AIDS Nursing Care in the Home. In *Nursing Care of the Person with AIDS/ARC*, ed. A. Lewis, 215–37. Rockville, Md.: Aspen.

Douglas, S., C. Kalman, and T. Kalman. 1985. Homophobia among Physicians and Nurses: An Empirical Study. *Hospital and Community Psychiatry* 36:1309–11.

Durham, J.D., and F.L. Cohen. 1987. *The Person with AIDS: Nursing Perspectives.* New York: Springer.

Fahrner, R. 1988. Nursing Interventions. In *Nursing Care of the Person with AIDS/ARC,* ed. A. Lewis, 115–30. Rockville, Md.: Aspen.

Friedman, S.R., D.C. Des Jarlais, J.L. Sothern, J. Garber, H. Cohen, and D. Smith. 1987. AIDS and Self-organization among Intravenous Drug Users. *International Journal of the Addictions* 22:201–19.

Gaut, D.A. 1979. An Application of the Kerr-Soltis Model to the Concept of Caring in Nursing Education. Ph.D. diss., College of Education, University of Washington, Seattle.

Green, K.C. 1987. The Talent Pool in Nursing: A Comparative and Longitudinal Perspective. *American Journal of Nursing* 87:1610–15.

Gross, J. 1988. Mission of an AIDS Unit Is Not to Cure, but to Care. *New York Times,* August 22.

Heron, E. 1988. *Intensive Care: The Story of a Nurse.* New York: Ivy Books/ Ballantine Books.

Institute of Medicine. 1983. *Study of Nursing.* Washington: National Academy Press.

Journal of Palliative Care. 1988. Special Issue on AIDS. 4 (4).

Kramer, M., and L. Hafner. 1989. Shared Values: Impact on Staff Nurse Job Satisfaction and Perceived Productivity. *Nursing Research* 38:172–77.

Kramer, M., and C. Schmalenberg. 1988. Magnet Hospitals: Institutions of Excellence. *Journal of Nursing Administration* 18:11–19.

Lambert, B. 1989. AIDS Patients Seen Straining Hospitals. *New York Times,* March 3.

Leininger, M.M. 1980. Caring: A Central Focus of Nursing and Health Care Services. *Nursing and Health Care* 1:135–43.

———. 1984. *Care: The Essence of Nursing and Health.* Thorofare, N.J.: Slack, Inc.

Lewis, A. 1988. The Community Provider Experience. In *Nursing Care of the Person with AIDS/ARC,* ed. A. Lewis, 307. Rockville, Md.: Aspen.

Maslach, C., and S.E. Jackson. 1982. Burnout in the Health Professions. In *Social Psychology of Health and Illness,* ed. G. Saunders and J. Suls, 79–103. Hillsdale, N.J.: Lawrence Erlbaum Associates.

Memorial Sloan-Kettering Cancer Center. No date. Standard Care Plan for the Patient with AIDS. New York.

Mayeroff, M. 1971. *On Caring.* New York: Harper and Row.

Morrison, C. 1987. Establishing a Therapeutic Environment: Institutional Resources. In *The Person with AIDS: Nursing Perspectives,* ed. J.D. Durham and F.L. Cohen, 110–24. New York: Springer.

———. 1988. Foreword. In *Nursing Care of the Person with AIDS/ ARC,* ed. A. Lewis, xviii–ix. Rockville, Md.: Aspen.

Moses, E.B. 1989. *Selected Findings from the 1988 Sample Survey of Regis-*

tered Nurses. Washington: U.S. Department of Health and Human Services, HRSA, Division of Nursing.

National Commission on Nursing. 1983. *Summary Report and Recommendations*. Chicago: Hospital Research and Educational Trust.

Peabody, B. 1986. *The Screaming Room: A Mother's Journal of Her Son's Struggle with AIDS: A True Story of Love, Dedication and Courage*. San Diego: Oak Tree.

Presidential Commission on the Human Immunodeficiency Virus Epidemic. 1988. *Report to the President*. Washington.

Reverby, S.M. 1987. *Ordered to Care: The Dilemma of American Nursing, 1850–1945*. New York: Cambridge University Press.

San Francisco General Hospital Nursing Staff. 1986. Nursing Care Plan for Persons with AIDS. *Quality Review Bulletin* 12:261–65.

Taravella, S. 1989. Reserving a Place to Treat AIDS Patients in the Hospital. *Modern Healthcare* 19:32–39.

Theis, E.C. 1986. Ethical Issues: A Nursing Perspective. *New England Journal of Medicine* 315:1222–24.

Tisdale, S. 1986. *The Sorcerer's Apprentice: Inside the Modern Hospital*. New York: McGraw Hill.

U.S. Department of Health and Human Services. 1988. *Secretary's Commission on Nursing: Final Report*. Washington.

van Servellen, G.M., C.E. Lewis, and B. Leake. 1988a. Nurses' Responses to the AIDS Crisis: Implications for Continuing Education Programs. *Journal of Continuing Education in Nursing* 19:4–8.

————. 1988b. Nurses' Knowledge, Attitudes and Fears about AIDS. *Journal of Nursing Science and Practice* 1:1–7.

Volberding, P.A. 1985. The Clinical Spectrum of the Acquired Immunodeficiency Syndrome: Implications for Comprehensive Patient Care. *Annals of Internal Medicine* 103:729–32.

Watson, J. 1979. *Nursing: The Philosophy and Science of Caring*. Boston: Little, Brown.

————. 1985. *Nursing: Human Science and Human Care*. Norwalk, Conn.: Appleton-Century-Crofts.

Wertz, D.C., J.R. Sorenson, L. Liebling, L. Kessler, and T.C. Heeren. 1987. Knowledge and Attitudes of AIDS Health Care Providers before and after Education Programs. *Public Health Reports* 102:248–54.

Witcher, G. 1987. Last Class of Nurses Told: Don't Stop Caring. (*Boston Globe*, May 13, 1985.) In *Ordered to Care: The Dilemma of American Nursing, 1859–1945*, ed. S.M. Reverby, 1. New York: Cambridge University Press.

Wolf, Z.R. 1988. *Nurses' Work: The Sacred and the Profane*. Philadelphia: University of Pennsylvania Press.

World Health Organization in collaboration with the International Council of Nurses. 1988. *Guidelines for Nursing Management of People Infected with Human Immunodeficiency Virus (HIV)*. Geneva: World Health Organization.

Worth, C. 1988. Handle With Care. *New York Times Magazine* (September 25): 60–62.

Acknowledgments: The drafting of this chapter was supported in part by a grant to Linda H. Aiken from the SmithKline Beckman Foundation. We would particularly like to thank JoAnne Bennett, a team nurse with the Gay Men's Health Crisis and a consultant/administrator in their educational and client services departments, and Donald Smith, clinical supervisor of the designated AIDS unit in Mt. Sinai Hospital, New York City, for sharing their first-hand AIDS nursing experience with us.

AIDS and its Impact on Medical Work
The Culture and Politics of the Shop Floor

CHARLES L. BOSK and JOEL E. FRADER

IN 1979 WHEN UNDERGRADUATES APPLIED IN RECORD numbers for admission to medical school, AIDS was not a clinical and diagnostic category. In 1990 when the applications to medical schools are plummeting, AIDS is unarguably with us, and not just as a clinical entity. AIDS has become what the French anthropologist Marcel Mauss called a "total social phenomenon—one whose transactions are at once economic, juridical, moral, aesthetic, religious and mythological, and whose meaning cannot, therefore, be adequately described from the point of view of any single discipline" (Hyde 1979). For cultural analysts, present and future, the 1980s and beyond are the AIDS years.

This chapter is about the impact of AIDS on the shop floor of the academic urban hospital, an attempt to understand the impact of AIDS on everyday practices of doctors providing inpatient care. Following Mauss, we wish to view AIDS as a total social phenomenon rather than as a mere disease. Procedurally, we shall concentrate on the house officer (someone who, after graduation from medical school, participates in medical specialty training) and the medical student to see how this new infectious disease changes the content of everyday work and the education of apprentice physicians learning how to doctor and to assume the social responsibilities of the role of the physician. We are going to look at professional and occupational culture as a set of shop-floor practices and beliefs about work.

At the close of this article we will make some generalizations about the impact of AIDS on medical training and reflect on how this affects the professional culture of physicians. This may distort the picture somewhat, as the urban teaching hospital is not representative of the whole world of medical practice. To the degree that AIDS patients are concentrated in them, any inferences drawn from large teaching hospitals overstate or exaggerate the impact of AIDS. At the very least, such sampling fails to catalogue the variety of strategies individual physicians may use to avoid patients with AIDS. It fails, as well, to capture the innovative approaches to AIDS of pioneering health professionals (many of whom also happen to be gay) in nontraditional settings.

This sampling problem notwithstanding, the urban academic teaching hospital is the arena of choice for studying the impact of AIDS on the medical profession. The concentration of cases in urban teaching hospitals means that students and house officers have a high likelihood of treating patients with AIDS. They are the physicians on the clinical front lines, the ones with the heaviest day-to-day operational burdens.

Further, our attention to the house officers and students possesses a secondary benefit for this inquiry into shop-floor or work-place culture: namely, the natural state of the work place in its before-AIDS condition has been extensively documented. We use the terms shop-floor and work-place culture to invoke the sociological tradition for inquiries into work begun by Everett C. Hughes (1971) at the University of Chicago in the post-World War II years. This tradition emphasizes equivalencies between humble and proud occupations, the management of "dirty work," the procedures that surround routines and emergencies, and the handling of mistakes. Above all, the perspective invites us to reverse our "conventional sentimentality" (Becker 1967) about occupations. The idea of the hospital as a shop floor is one rhetorical device for reminding us that house officers and students are workers in a very real and active sense.

Numerous autobiographical accounts beginning with the pseudonymous Dr. X of *Intern*, catalogue the conditions of the shop floor (Dr. X. 1965; a partial list of subsequent narratives includes Nolen 1970; Rubin 1972; Sweeney 1973; Bell 1975; Haseltine and Yaw 1976; Horowitz and Offen 1977; Mullan 1976; Morgan 1980). There have also been similar commentaries on medical schools (Le Baron 1981;

Klass 1987; Klein 1981; Konner 1987; Reilly 1987). Novels by former
house officers have also described the work-place culture of physicians
in training and the tensions inherent in it. (Examples of this genre include Cook 1972; Glasser 1973; and Shem 1978.)

In addition, there is a large literature on the socialization of medical
students and house officers; each of these can be viewed as studies of
shop-floor culture. (For a critical overview of this literature see Bosk
1985; individual studies of note include Fox 1957; Fox and Lief 1963;
Becker et al. 1961; and Coombs 1978.) The literature on house officers
is even more extensive. (See Mumford 1970 and Miller 1970 on medical internships; Mizrahi 1986 on internal medicine residencies; Light
1980 and Coser 1979 on psychiatry; Scully 1980 on obstetrics and gynecology; and Bosk 1979 and Milman 1976 on surgery; Burkett and Knafl
1976 on orthopedic surgeons; and Stelling and Bucher 1972 have focused on how house officers either avoid or accept monitoring by
superordinates.)

We can construct a before-AIDS shop-floor culture as a first step in
assessing what difference AIDS makes in the occupational culture of
physicians. Our picture of the after-AIDS shop floor arises from the
pictures drawn in the medical literature, our teaching and consulting
experience in large university health centers, and 30 interviews with
medical personnel caring for AIDS patients in ten teaching hospitals.
These interviews were conducted with individuals at all levels of training and provide admittedly impressionistic data, which need more systematic verification. The interviews averaged an hour in length and
explored both how workers treated AIDS patients and how they felt
about the patients.

Shop-floor Culture before AIDS: Exploitation and Powerlessness

The pre-AIDS shop floor in academic medical centers is not a particularly happy place, as depicted in first-hand accounts of medical education. The dominant tone of many of the volumes is a bitter cynicism,
captured in two of the dedications: Glasser's work is "For all the Ar-
rowsmiths"; Cook dedicates his volume "to the ideal of medicine we all

held the year we entered medical school." The set of everyday annoyances extends considerably beyond the long hours of work, although these alone are burdensome. Beyond that there is the fact that much of the work is without any profit for the house officer; it is "scut" work, essential drudgery whose completion appears to add little to the worker's overall sense of mastery and competence. (Becker et al. 1961 first commented that medical students, like their more senior trainees, disliked tasks that neither allowed them to exercise medical responsibility nor increased their clinical knowledge.) Consider here a resident's reaction to a day in the operating room, assisting on major surgery:

I urinated, wrote all the preoperative orders, changed my clothes, and had some dinner, in that order. As I walked across to the dining room, I felt as if I'd been run over by a herd of wild elephants in heat. I was exhausted and, much worse, deeply frustrated. I'd been assisting in surgery for nine hours. Eight of them had been the most important in Mrs. Takura's [a patient] life; yet I felt no sense of accomplishment. I had simply endured, and I was probably the one person they could have done without. Sure, they needed retraction, but a catatonic schizophrenic would have sufficed. Interns are eager to work hard, even to sacrifice—above all, to be useful and to display their special talents—in order to learn. I felt none of these satisfactions, only an empty bitterness and exhaustion (Cook 1972, 74).

The complaint is not atypical.

In all accounts, house officers and students complain about the ways their energies are wasted because they are inundated with scut work of various types. If procedures are to be done on time, house officers have to act as a back-up transport service. If test results are to be interpreted and patients diagnosed, then house officers have to track down the results; they are their own messenger service. In many hospitals house officers and students do the routine venipunctures and are responsible for maintaining the intravenous lines of patients requiring them. Routine bloodwork composes a large amount of the physician-in-training's everyday scut work.

Their inability to control either their own or their patients' lives, their fundamental powerlessness, and the exploitation of their labors by the "greedy" institution (Coser 1979) that is the modern academic hospital are all at the center of physicians' accounts of their training.

Clinical Coups and Defeats

The juxtaposition of labors that are both Herculean and pointless account for the major narrative themes in accounts of patient care. First, there are stories of "clinical coups." These are dramatic instances where the house officer's labors were not pointless, where a tricky diagnostic problem was solved and a timely and decisive intervention to save a life was initiated. Such stories are rare but all the house officer accounts, even the most bitter, tell at least one. These tales reinforce—even in the face of the contradictory details of the rest of the narrative—that the house officer's efforts make a difference, however small; that the pain and suffering of both doctors and patients are not invariably pointless; and that professional heroism may still yield a positive result, even if only rarely.

More numerous by far in the narratives are accounts of "clinical defeats." A few of these tales concern the apprentice physician's inability to come to the right decision quickly enough; these are personal defeats. The bulk of these tales, however, concern defeat (indexed by death) even though all the right things were done medically. Narratives of clinical defeats generally emphasize the tension in the conflict between care and cure, between quantity and quality of life, between acting as a medical scientist and acting as a human being.

The repeated accounts of clinical defeats reinforce at one level the general pointlessness of much of the house officers' effort. They recount situations in which house officers either are too overwhelmed to provide clinical care or in which the best available care does not ensure a favorable outcome. But the stories of defeat tell another tale as well. Here, house officers describe how they learn that despite the failings of their technical interventions they can make a difference, that care is often more important than cure, and that the human rewards of their medical role are great. Each of the first-hand accounts of medical training features a tale of defeat that had a transformative effect on the physician in training. Each tale of defeat encodes a lesson about the psychological growth of the human being shrouded in the white coat of scientific authority. For example, Glasser's *Ward 402* (1973) centers on the unexpected decline and death, following initial successful treatment, of an eleven-year-old girl with acute leukemia. The interaction with her angry, anxious, and oppositional parents and the futile medical struggle to overcome neurologic complications forces the protagonist to see beyond the narrow medical activism that he had been carefully taught. In the end the intern hero literally pulls the plug on the child's respirator and goes off to see the angry, drunken father vowing, this time, to listen.

Psychological Detachment and Adolescent Invulnerability

The shop-floor culture of house officers and students is largely a peer culture. The senior authority of faculty appears absent, at best, or disruptive and intrusive, at worst, in the first-hand narratives of clinical training. That is to say, the clinical wisdom of faculty is unavailable when house officers need it; when clinical faculty are present, they "pimp" (humiliate by questioning) house officers during rounds with questions on obscure details or order them to perform mindless tasks easily performed by those (nurses, technicians) far less educated about the pathophysiology of disease.

As a result, house officers feel isolated and embattled. Patients, other staff, and attending faculty are the enemy; each is the source of a set of never-ending demands and ego-lacerating defeats. Konner (1987, 375), an anthropologist who acquired a medical degree, is quite eloquent on the theme of the patient as enemy:

> It is obvious from what I have written here that the stress of clinical training alienates the doctor from the patient, that in a real sense the patient becomes the enemy. (Goddamit did she blow her I.V. again? Jesus Christ did he spike a temp?) At first I believed that this was an inadvertent and unfortunate concomitant of medical training, but I now think that it is intrinsic. Not only stress and sleeplessness but the sense of the patient as the cause of one's distress contributes to the doctor's detachment. This detachment is not just objective but downright negative. To cut and puncture a person, to take his or her life in your hands, to pound the chest until ribs break, to decide upon drastic action without being able to ask permission, to render a judgment about whether care should continue or stop—these and a thousand other things may require something

stronger than objectivity. They may actually require a measure of dislike.

This sentiment is not, of course, unique to Konner. One sociologist, writing about the socialization process in internal medicine, found negative sentiments about patients so rife that she titled her account *Getting Rid of Patients* (Mizrahi 1986).

Feelings about patients are most visibly displayed in the slang that physicians in training use to describe patients. Beyond the well-known "Gomer" (George and Dundes 1978; Leiderman and Grisso 1985), there is a highly articulated language that refers to patients in distress. Along with the slang, there is much black and "gallows" humor. This black humor is a prominent feature of Shem's (1978) *House of God*.

The slang and humor highlight the psychological and social distance between patients and those who care for them medically. This distance is best exemplified in Shem's "Law IV" of the House of God: "The patient is the one with the disease." The reverse, of course, is that the doctor does not have a problem. He or she is invulnerable. In the first-hand accounts of training, physicians' feelings of invulnerability appear and reappear. The doctors treat disease but they are rarely touched by it (save for the occasional exemplary patient with whom physicians make a psychological connection). To these young apprentice physicians, disease is rarely, if ever, personally threatening and rarely, if ever, presented as something that could happen to the physician. (Many doctors reacted with shock to Lear's (1980) account of her urologist-husband's careless and callous treatment. These readers seemed to have assumed their M.D.s protected them somehow.) Moreover, given that hospitals (outside of pediatrics and before AIDS) housed a high proportion of patients substantially older than house officers, patterns of mortality and morbidity themselves reinforced the sense of invulnerability. It is the rare patient close in age to the author who provokes distress and introspection about doctoring on the part of writers of first-hand narratives.

The fantasy of invulnerability takes on an adolescent quality when one notes the cavalier tone used to describe some of life's most awful problems and the oppositional stance taken toward patients and attending faculty. There may be something structural in this; just as adolescence is betwixt and between childhood and adulthood, the

physician-in-training is likewise liminal, betwixt studenthood and professional independence.

The Coming of AIDS to the Shop Floor:
Risk and the Loss of Invulnerability

Before AIDS entered the shop floor, physicians in training had many
objections to work-place conditions. Not only that, AIDS entered a
shop floor that was in the process of transformation from major political, social, organizational, and economic policy changes regarding
health care. These changes have been elaborated in detail elsewhere
(Light 1980; Starr 1982; Relman 1980; Mechanic 1986) and need only
brief mention here. Acute illnesses, especially infectious diseases, have
given way to chronic disorders. The patient population has aged
greatly. There has been a relatively new public emphasis on individual
responsibility for one's medical problems—diet, smoking, nonther-
apeutic drug use, "excessive" alcohol use, exercise, etc. (Fox 1986).

Of great importance has been the redefinition of medical care as a
service *like any other* in the economy with individual medical decisions
subject to the kind of fiscal scrutiny applied to the purchase of au-
tomobiles or dry cleaning. Achieving reduced costs through shorter
hospitalizations and other measures, however, has created more intensive scheduling for those caring for patients on the hospital's wards—
even if the hospital's capacity shrinks in the name of efficiency. Fewer
patients are admitted to the hospital and they stay for shorter periods
of time, yet more things are done to and for them, increasing the
house officers' clerical, physical, and intellectual work while decreasing
the opportunity for trainees to get to know their patients (Rabkin
1982; Steiner et al. 1987). The beds simply fill up with comparatively
sicker, less communicative patients who need more intensive care.

All the shifts in the medical care system have changed the reality of
hospital practice in ways that may not conform to the expectations of
those entering the medical profession. In addition to the usual disillu-
sionment occurring in training, the contemporary urban teaching hospital brings fewer opportunities for hope (Glick 1988). To the extent
that AIDS contributes to the population of more desperately ill
hospitalized patients, it exacerbates house officers' feelings of exploita-

tion and, because of its fatal outcome, AIDS adds to their sense of powerlessness. We must assess the impact of AIDS against this background of old resentments and new burdens.

AIDS has certainly not improved the work climate of the medical shop floor. The most apparent phenomenon related to AIDS in the contemporary urban teaching hospital is risk or, more precisely, the *perception* of risk. The orthodox medical literature proclaims, over and over, that the AIDS virus does not pass readily from patient to care giver (Lifson et al. 1986; Gerberding et al. 1987). But some medical writing dwells on risks (Gerbert et al. 1988; Becker, Cone, and Gerberding 1989; O'Connor 1990) and observations of behavior make clear that fear on the wards is rampant. Workers of all types, including doctors, have at times sheathed themselves in inappropriate armor or simply refused to approach the patients at all. Klass (1987, 185) put it quite starkly: "We have to face the fact that we are going through these little rituals of sanitary precaution partly because we are terrified of this disease and are not willing to listen to anything our own dear medical profession may tell us about how it actually is or is not transmitted."

Perceptions of risk can and do change with time and experience. Our interviewees and commentators in the literature indicate that as individuals and institutions have more patients with AIDS they begin to shed some of their protective garb. In one hospital we were told that the practice of donning gown, gloves, and masks became less frequent as doctors, nurses, housekeepers, and dietary workers "saw" that they did not get AIDS from their patients. This, of course, raises another interesting question: In what sense did personnel come to this conclusion? After all, the diseases associated with HIV infection typically have long latencies, up to several years, before symptoms develop. None of the institutions where our informants worked conducted routine surveillance to assess development of HIV antibody among personnel. Thus, staff could not really know if they had "gotten" HIV infection. Moreover, reports of individual physicians anxiously awaiting the results of HIV tests after needle sticks have now become a staple of the oral culture of academic medical centers.

On AIDS wards all personnel are far less likely to place barriers between themselves and patients for activities where blood or other body fluids might be transmitted. Beyond subspecialty units, however, medical, nursing, and support staff are far more fearful and employ many more nonrational techniques to prevent contamination. (We refer to simple touching, as in noninvasive patient examinations, back rubs, etc., as well as activities involving no patient contact at all, such as the placing of meal trays on overbed tables or sweeping the floor.) One informant told us that HIV-infected hemophilia patients in one hospital often refuse hospitalization if it means getting a room on certain floors or nursing units. The patients prefer to delay needed treatment until a bed becomes available on a unit where they feel more humanely treated.

Several other curious phenomena have emerged regarding risks and AIDS in the medical work place. While in some locations lack of experience has led to classic reactions of fear and avoidance, in other places the paucity of experience permits denial to dominate. The comments of house staff in a hospital with only an occasional AIDS patient indicated that few residents followed Centers for Disease Control or similar guidelines for "universal precautions." Various explanations were offered, including the conviction that starting intravenous infusions, blood drawing, or similar procedures is more difficult when wearing gloves. When asked how surgeons accomplish complex manual tasks while wearing one or two pairs of gloves, residents usually replied that they had not learned to do things "that way." Here, one kind of inexperience (with gloves) reinforces another (with AIDS), bolstering the feeling of invulnerability that was widespread before AIDS.

Some medical students and physicians have dealt with the problem of risk globally. They want to avoid encountering patients with AIDS altogether. In one medical school where we teach, there is a policy prohibiting students from refusing to care for HIV-infected patients. The policy infuriates many students, a fact we learned in medical-ethics discussion groups that met to discuss an AIDS case. They cited several reasons. The rules, some felt, were changed midstream. Had they known about the policy, they might have chosen another school. They felt they had no role in the formation of the policy and that the tremendous economic investment they made in the institution, in the form of tuition, entitles them to some decision-making authority. They objected to the rule's existence. They said such rules have no place in medicine. Doctors, they believe, should have as much freedom as lawyers, accountants, executives, or others to accept or reject "clients" or "customers." When presented with the notion of a professional obligation or duty, based upon generally acknowledged moral precepts, they balked. At other institutions we know there has been more controversy among medical students, with some making impassioned statements about the physician's obligation to treat. In this debate we see AIDS as a total social phenomenon acting as a vehicle for debating and defining standards of professional conduct.

Another aspect of medical risk avoidance may be revealed through the changing patterns of residency selection. For some time there has been a shift away from primary care specialities like internal medicine, family practice, and pediatrics toward specialities such as orthopedics, ophthalmology, otolaryngology, and radiology (McCarty 1987). The reasons for this phenomena are not entirely clear, but include the technical, rather than personal, orientation of the medical training system and the higher compensation available in the latter group of specialties, sought, in part, because of staggering educational debts. In the past few years, the trend may have accelerated, with internal medicine (whose house staff and practitioners provide the bulk of the care for AIDS patients) training programs failing to find sufficient qualified applicants (Graettianger 1989; Davidoff 1989). This crisis has been most marked in the cities with large numbers of HIV-infected patients (Ness et al. 1989). A similar trend toward avoiding residencies in AIDS endemic areas may be emerging in pediatrics, according to faculty rumors; a substantial proportion of pediatric house officers, like those in internal medicine, would not care for AIDS patients if given the choice, according to one survey (Link et al. 1988). (This does not imply that defenses such as denial and risk avoidance were not part of the medical educational culture prior to AIDS. Indeed, denial is at the center of the syndrome of adolescent invulnerability. Distinctive now is the appearance of such sentiments in professional journals.)

Surgical Risk and Historical Precedent

Even more remarkable in the AIDS-risk reaction has been the appearance in prestigious medical journals of complaints, whines, and pleas for understanding from doctors worried about contamination and ruination (Guy 1987; Ponsford 1987; Dudley and Sim 1988; Carey 1988; Guido 1988). These pieces offer various estimates of risk to person, career, family, future patients deprived of the skills of the author or his or her esteemed colleagues, and other justifications for not treating

HIV-infected persons. (At last, the attending authors may have forged an alliance with their house officers by championing the cause of self-protection.) The articles proclaim a kind of anticoup, that is, they are declarations of futility, contrasting sharply with the verbal swaggering of pre-AIDS narratives. It is important to note that the medical literature on AIDS is not entirely negative; complaints can be matched against calls to duty (Gillon 1987; Zuger and Miles 1987; Pellegrino 1987; Kim and Perfect 1988; Friedland 1988; Emanuel 1988; Sharp 1988; Peterson 1989). On the shop floor and in the literature, AIDS as a total social phenomenon has become the lens for focusing on the obligations of members of the medical profession.

Surgeons have been particularly outspoken about the extent to which they are threatened, and there *is* reason for their special concerns (Hagen, Meyer, and Pauker 1988; Peterson 1989). After all, these doctors have a high likelihood of contact with the blood of patients. This involves not just working in blood-perfused tissues, but also a risk of having gloves and skin punctured by the instruments of their craft or having blood splash onto other vulnerable areas of the body (mucous membranes in professional parlance). Surgeons, by the very nature of their work, do more of this than many other doctors. But other physicians do find themselves in similar circumstances, depending on their activities. Intensive-care specialists, invasive cardiologists, emergency physicians, pulmonary and gastrointestinal specialists, and others have frequent and/or sustained contact with the blood or other body fluids of patients who may be infected with HIV. House staff, as the foot soldiers doing comprehensive examinations, drawers of blood specimens, inserters of intravenous catheters or other tubes in other places, cleaners of wounds, or simply as those first on the scene of bloody disasters, are particularly likely to be splashed, splattered, or otherwise coated with patients' blood, secretions, or excretions.

We do not have data on the extent to which fears have or have not been translated into changes in behavior in operating and/or procedure rooms. In some communities there may now be fewer operations and these procedures may take longer as extra time is taken to reduce bleeding and avoid punctures. This may not turn out to be as good as it might at first seem. To the extent that high-risk patients have operations delayed or denied or must undergo longer anesthetics and have wounds open longer, patient care may be compromised.

It is interesting to compare the current outcry with what happened when medical science discovered the nature of hepatitis and recognized the medical risks to personnel of serum hepatitis, now known as hepatitis B. As long ago as 1949 (Liebowitz et al. 1949), the medical literature acknowledged that medical personnel coming in contact with blood stood at risk from hepatitis. A debate continued through the 1950s, 1960s, and early 1970s about whether surgeons were especially vulnerable because of their use of sharp instruments, the frequency of accidental puncture of the skin during surgical procedures, and the likelihood of inoculation of the virus into the bloodstream of the wounded party. The risks were felt to be clearly documented in an article (Rosenberg et al. 1973) in the *Journal of the American Medical Association* that commented: "This study demonstrates the distinct occupational hazard to surgeons when they operate on patients who are capable of transmitting hepatitis virus. . . . We believe that serious attempts should be made to prevent future epidemics. . . . Education and constant vigilance in surgical technique are central to any preventive program." Nowhere does the article suggest surgeons should consider not operating on patients at risk for hepatitis.

Of course, hepatitis B is not associated with a fatal prognosis in a large proportion of cases and is not entirely comparable to AIDS. Nonetheless, the epidemiologic evidence gathered in the 1970s suggested that hepatitis B was very prevalent among physicians, especially surgeons (Denes et al. 1978), and that medical personnel seemed especially vulnerable to having severe courses of the disease (Garibaldi et al. 1973). A portion become chronic carriers of the virus, with the added risk later of liver cancer and liver failure from cirrhosis. Moreover, secondary spread from infected medical workers can occur to patients (through small cuts and sores on the workers' skin) and sexual partners (through exchange of bodily fluids). Despite all this, major medical journals did not carry discussions of whether doctors at risk might be excused from professional activities. It may be that our society's general risk aversiveness (Fairlie 1989) and tolerance of self-centeredness have escalated sufficiently to make public renunciation of professional responsibility more acceptable. More likely, the general medical professional ethic has changed to one closer to that of the entrepreneur, as was true for our students. But perhaps something else is going on that, being synergistic with the perceived loss of invulnerability brought on by AIDS, makes the AIDS era distinctive.

AIDS as a Total Social Phenomenon

The reaction to AIDS on the shop floor must be examined in light of the perceptions of risk, the epidemiology of AIDS, and moral judgments some make about activities that lead to acquiring the disease. Most AIDS patients have come from identifiable populations: the gay community, intravenous drug users and their partners, and those who have gotten the disease from medical use of blood and blood products. While hepatitis B infections were prevalent in these populations and also entailed risks to medical personnel, hepatitis in such patients did not cause doctors to deny their professional responsibility to provide treatment. We are arguing that the unique combination of factors associated with AIDS prompts the negative reactions among doctors: changing tolerances of risk, the shift to an occupation bounded by entrepreneurial rules rather than professional duties, a specific fear of the terrible outcome should one acquire AIDS from a patient, objections to some of the specific behaviors that lead to AIDS, and class and racial bias. Below, we discuss some of the social characteristics of AIDS patients that affect the negativity of the professionals.

The demographics of AIDS is striking and flies rudely in the face of the last several decades of medical progress. Most AIDS patients are young adults. This is true of gays, drug users, and even the hemophiliacs, by and large. Most house officers, however naive and unprepared they are to confront devastating illness and death, at least have a general cultural and social expectation of, if not experience with, the death of old people. With AIDS, many of the sickest patients filling teaching hospital wards in high-prevalence cities are in their prime years, similar in age to the house staff providing the front-line care (Glick 1988). People so young are not supposed to die. These deaths challenge the ideology of the coming-if-not-quite-arrived triumph of modern medical science implicitly provided young doctors in medical education. (Two former house officers have written about the effects of AIDS on medical training: Wachter 1986; Zuger 1987.)

We do not want to paint with too broad a brush here. There are some important differences among the groups of AIDS patients, which influence the reactions of resident physicians. Our informants describe three nonexhaustive groups of patients to whom young doctors and students react: hemophiliacs and others who acquired AIDS through transfusion, young gay men, and drug users and their partners. (We have insufficient information to comment on the reaction to the rapidly growing infant AIDS population. Also, we cannot fully assess how attitudes toward any of these groups may have changed from the pre-AIDS era. Clearly, some in the health care system treated gays and IV drug users badly before they perceived a threat from them.)

In many ways, the patients who develop AIDS from blood products constitute a simple set. These patients are clearly seen as innocents, true victims of unfortunate but inevitable delay between recognition of a technical problem — blood-borne transmission of a serious disease — and its reliable and practical prevention — cleaning up of the blood supply. A chief resident commented that her house officers talk differently about patients with AIDS caused by transfusions from the way they speak about other AIDS patients. "The residents see these cases [with blood-product-related disease] as more tragic; their hearts go out to them more." Hemophiliacs have an air of double tragedy about them: an often crippling, always inconvenient genetic disorder made worse as a direct consequence of their medical treatment.

Hemophiliac patients with AIDS in one of the hospitals where we made inquiries went out of their way to make the origins of their disease or other emblems of their identity known. These patients "display" wives and children to differentiate themselves from homosexual patients. One hemophiliac, reflecting on his desire to have others know that his HIV-positive status preceded his drug abuse, commented that this public knowledge was important because there is "always a pecking order" in who gets scarce nursing care. Even though few people hold these patients in any way responsible for their disease, behavior on the wards toward HIV-positive hemophiliacs clearly differs from attention given non-AIDS or non-HIV-infected patients. As mentioned earlier, their hospital rooms are not as clean as the rooms of hemophiliac patients not infected with HIV; the staff does not touch them as often as they once did. (Many of these patients were frequently hospitalized before the HIV epidemic; in effect, they have served as their own controls in a cruel experiment of nature.) Their care is compromised in small but painful ways.

Gay patients with AIDS occupy an intermediate position in the hierarchy. The social characteristics of many of these patients, in the eyes of our informants, were positive ones: the patients were well educated, well groomed, took an active interest in their treatments, had supportive family and/or networks that relieved some of the burdens from their care providers, and the like. Of course, not all medical personnel appreciate all of these features. Interest in care has emerged into social activism about treatment, which some physicians resent. For example, one patient who had developed severe difficulty swallowing, and was starving as a consequence, requested insertion of a feeding tube through his abdominal wall into his intestinal tract. His primary physicians tried to put him off, apparently believing he would succumb soon, no matter what was done. When he persisted, a surgical consultant was called. The surgeon initially treated the request as a joke, finally agreed after an attempt to dissuade the patient ("So, you really want to do this?"), and then provided no follow-up care. This is but one case, but our general impression is that the "turfing" (transferring) that Shem (1978) described as a major feature of shop-floor culture before AIDS has intensified. Physicians want to shift the burdens and responsibilities of care to others.

From the resident's point of view, there may also be a down side to the extensive support systems many gay patients enjoy. In the final stages of AIDS, little more can be done for patients beyond providing comfort. For the interested and compassionate resident, titration of pain medication and less technical interaction, that is, talking with the patient, can be therapeutic for both. If the patient has become invested in alternative treatments for discomfort, from herbal medicine to meditation to imaging, and if the patient is surrounded by loving family and community, the house officer may feel she or he has nothing whatsoever to contribute. This helplessness amplifies the despair and the pointlessness of whatever scut work must be done. Here, there can be no transforming, heroic intervention, no redemption arising from clinical defeat.

The IV-drug-using HIV-infected patients represent one of the fastest growing and most problematic set of patients. Teaching hospitals have always had more than their share of patients who are "guilty" victims of disease, that is, patients whose medical problems are seen as direct consequences of their behavior. Many of our prestigious teaching hospitals have been municipal or county facilities filled with substance-abusing patients with a wide spectrum of problems from which house staff have learned. Our informants suggested that the coming of AIDS to this population had subtly altered the way these patients are regarded. Now, drug users cannot be regarded with mere contempt or simple disrespect: there is fear among doctors who are afraid of acquiring AIDS from the patients. Whereas frustration and anger in some cases (especially when drug users were manipulative or physically threatening) and indifference in others used to constitute much of the response to drug-using patients, fear of AIDS has added a difficult dimension.

One might argue that before HIV, this underclass population had a set of positive social roles to play. Their very presence reminded doctors and nurses, perhaps even other patients, that things might not be as bad as they seemed. The intern might be miserable after staying up an entire weekend, but she/he could look to a better life ahead and know that she/he did not have to face homelessness and desperate poverty when finally leaving the hospital to rest. Moreover, the underclass patients provided chances to learn and practice that private patients could not offer. (The poor often have more complex or advanced medical problems, compared with wealthier patients, because of limited access to care and delays in diagnosis and treatment. In addition, attendings often permit house staff to exercise greater responsibility with "service" patients.) But AIDS seems to have changed the balance for many who might have tolerated or welcomed the opportunities to care for the underserved. For a medical student contemplating a residency, what was previously a chance to gain relative autonomy quickly in an institution with many substance-abusing patients may have become predominantly unwelcome exposure to a dreadful illness. If this is so, AIDS will trigger, in yet another way, a dreadful decline in the availability and quality of care for America's medical underclass.

Conclusion

The full impact of AIDS on the modern system of medical care will not be clear for many years. Nevertheless, the disease has already affected the culture of American medicine in a pivotal place: the urban teaching center. Already a scene beset with anger, pain, sadness, and high technology employed soullessly against disease, AIDS has added to the troubles. We cannot know for certain whether this new plague has contributed to the decline in interest in medicine as a career or to the flight from primary care. There is certainly no evidence that AIDS has prompted many to seek out a life of selfless dedication to tending the hopelessly ill.

For those who have chosen to train in hospitals with large numbers of AIDS patients, the disease has added to the burdens of the shop floor. The perception of risk of acquiring AIDS has undermined one of the best-established defenses house officers have relied on: the maintenance of an air of invulnerability. Some doctors are so scared they are abandoning their traditional duty and no longer seem able or willing to try to bring off the heroic coup against daunting clinical odds. To be sure, this fear is fed by other factors on the social scene: the economic changes in medicine, transforming the profession into the province of the entrepreneur; the youth and other characteristics of many AIDS patients; and the willingness of the entire society to turn away from the underclass, especially from those who are seen as self-destructive.

Nothing here suggests that AIDS will spark a turn to a kinder, gentler medical care system. Those in the educational system inclined to seek models providing compassionate medical care will likely find few attractive mentors. Instead, they will meet burned-out martyrs, steely-eyed technicians, and teachers filled with fear. Tomorrow's first-hand accounts of medical education and fictionalized autobiographies may, as a result, be even grimmer than yesterday's.

There is the possibility that this conclusion is too stark, too depressing. For those desperate for a more hopeful scenario, at least one other alternative suggests itself. As the numbers of medical students dwindle, perhaps those who enter will be more committed to ideals of professional service and, among those, some will enter with a missionary zeal for caring for AIDS patients. There is little to suggest this other than the portraits of the few heroic physicians one finds in Shilts's (1987) account of the early years of the AIDS epidemic. If these physicians inspire a new generation of medical professionals, then the tone of future first-hand accounts will be more in line with the highest ideals and aspirations of the medical profession.

References

Becker, H. 1967. Whose Side Are We On? *Social Problems* 14:239–47.

Becker, C.E., J.E. Cone and J. Gerberding. 1989. Occupational Infection with Human Immunodeficiency Virus (HIV): Risks and Risk Reduction. *Annals of Internal Medicine* 110:653–56.

Becker, H., B. Geer, E.C. Hughes, and A. Strauss. 1961. *Boys in White: Student Culture in Medical School*. Chicago: University of Chicago Press.

Bell, D. 1975. *A Time To Be Born*. New York: Dell.

Bosk, C. 1979. *Forgive and Remember: Managing Medical Failure.* Chicago: University of Chicago Press.

————. 1985. Social Controls and Physicians: The Oscillation of Cynicism and Idealism in Sociological Theory. In *Social Controls and the Medical Profession*, ed. J.P. Swazey and S.R. Scherr, 31–52. Boston: Oelgeschlager, Gunn and Hain.

Burkett, G., and K. Knafl. 1974. Judgment and Decision-making in a Medical Specialty. *Sociology of Work and Occupations* 1:82-109.

Carey, J.S. 1988. Routine Preoperative Screening for HIV (Letter to the Editor). *Journal of the American Medical Association* 260:179.

Cook, R. 1972. *The Year of the Intern.* New York: Harcourt Brace Jovanovich.

Coombs, R.H. 1978. *Mastering Medicine: Professional Socialization of Medical School.* New York: Free Press.

Coser, L. 1974. *Greedy Institutions: Patterns of Undivided Commitment.* New York: Free Press.

Coser, R.L. 1979. *Training in Ambiguity: Learning through Doing in a Mental Hospital.* New York: Free Press.

Davidoff, F. 1989. Medical Residencies: Quantity or Quality? *Annals of Internal Medicine* 110:757-58.

Denes, A.E., J.L. Smith, J.E. Maynard, I.L. Doto, K.R. Berquist, and A.J. Finkel. 1978. Hepatitis B Infection in Physicians: Results of a Nationwide Seroepidemiologic Survey. *Journal of the American Medical Association* 239:210-12.

Dudley, H.A.F., and A. Sim. 1988. AIDS: A Bill of Rights for the Surgical Team? *British Medical Journal* 296:1449-50.

Emanuel, E.J. 1988. Do Physicians Have an Obligation to Treat Patients with AIDS? *New England Journal of Medicine* 318:1686-90.

Fairlie, H. 1989. Fear of Living: America's Morbid Aversion to Risk. *New Republic* January 23:14-19.

Fox, D. 1986. AIDS and the American Health Polity: The History and Prospects of a Crisis of Authority. *Milbank Quarterly* 64 (suppl. 1):7-33.

Fox, R.C. 1957. Training for Uncertainty. In *The Student-Physician: Introductory Studies in the Sociology of Medical Education*, ed. R.K. Merton, G.C. Reader, and P.L. Kendall, 207-41. Cambridge: Harvard University Press.

Fox, R.C., and H. Lief. 1963. Training for "Detached Concern" in Medical Students. In *The Psychological Basis of Medical Practice*, ed. H. Lief, V. Lief, and N. Lief, 12-35. New York: Harper and Row.

Friedland, G. 1988. AIDS and Compassion. *Journal of the American Medical Association* 259:2898-99.

Garibaldi, R.A., J.N. Forrest, J.A. Bryan, B.F. Hanson, and W.E. Dismukes. 1973. Hemodialysis-Associated Hepatitis. *Journal of the American Medical Association* 225:384-89.

George, V., and A. Dundes. 1978. The Gomer: A Figure of American Hospital Folk Speech. *Journal of American Folklore* 91:568-81.

Gerberding, J.L., C.E. Bryant-LeBlanc, K. Nelson, A.R. Moss, D. Osmond, H.F. Chambers, J.R. Carlson, W.L. Drew, J.A. Levy, and M.A. Sande. 1987. Risk of Transmitting the Human Immunodeficiency Virus, Cytomegalovirus, and Hepatitis B Virus to Health Care Workers Exposed to Patients with AIDS and AIDS-related Conditions. *Journal of Infectious Diseases* 156:1-8.

Gerbert, B., B. Maguire, V. Badner, D. Altman, and G. Stone. 1988. Why Fear Persists: Health Care Professionals and AIDS. *Journal of the American Medical Association* 260:3481-83.

Gillon, R. 1987. Refusal to Treat AIDS and HIV Positive Patients. *British Medical Journal* 294:1332-33.

Glasser, R.J. 1973. *Ward 402*. New York: George Braziller.

Glick, S.M. 1988. The Impending Crisis in Internal Medicine Training Programs. *American Journal of Medicine* 84:929-32.

Graettinger, J.S. 1989. Internal Medicine in the National Resident Matching Program 1978-1989. *Annals of Internal Medicine* 110:682.

Guido, L.J. 1988. Routine Preoperative Screening for HIV (Letter to the Editor). *Journal of the American Medical Association* 260:180.

Guy, P.J. 1987. AIDS: A Doctor's Duty. *British Medical Journal* 294-445.

Hagen, M.D., K.B. Meyer, and S.G. Pauker. 1988. Routine Preoperative Screening for HIV: Does the Risk to the Surgeon Outweigh the Risk to the Patient? *Journal of the American Medical Association* 259:1357-59.

Haseltine, F., and Y. Yaw. 1976. *Woman Doctor: The Internship of a Modern Woman*. Boston: Houghton Mifflin.

Horowitz, S., and N. Offen. 1977. *Calling Dr. Horowitz*. New York: William Morrow.

Hughes, E.C. 1971. *The Sociological Eye: Selected Papers on Work, Self, and Society*. Chicago: Aldine-Atherton.

Hyde, L. 1979. *The Gift: Imagination and the Erotic Life of Property*. New York: Vintage Books.

Kim, J.H., and J.R. Perfect. 1988. To Help the Sick: An Historical and Ethical Essay Concerning the Refusal to Care for Patients with AIDS. *American Journal of Medicine* 84:135-38.

Klass, P. 1987. *A Not Entirely Benign Procedure: Four Years as a Medical Student*. New York: Putnam.

Klein, K. 1981. *Getting Better: A Medical Student's Story*. Boston: Little, Brown.

Konner, M. 1987. *Becoming a Doctor: A Journey of Initiation in Medical School*. New York: Viking.

Lear, M.W. 1980. *Heartsounds*. New York: Pocket Books.

LeBaron, C. 1981. *Gentle Vengeance: An Account of the First Year at Harvard Medical School*. New York: Richard Marek.

Liebowitz, S., L. Greenwald, I. Cohen, and J. Litwins. 1949. Serum Hepatitis in a Blood Bank Worker. *Journal of the American Medical Association* 140(17):1331-33.

Leiderman, D., and J. Grisso. 1985. The Gomer Phenomenon. *Journal of Health and Social Behavior* 26:222-31.

Lifson, A.R., K.G. Castro, E. McCray, and H.W. Jaffe. 1986. National Surveillance of AIDS in Health Care Workers. *Journal of the American Medical Association* 265:3231-34.

Light, D. 1980. *Becoming Psychiatrists: The Professional Transformation of Self.* New York: W.W. Norton.

Link, R.N., A.R. Feingold, M.H. Charap, K. Freeman, and S.P. Shelov. 1988. Concerns of Medical and Pediatric House Officers about Acquiring AIDS from Their Patients. *American Journal of Public Health* 78:455-59.

McCarty, D.J. 1987. Why Are Today's Medical Students Choosing High-technology Specialties over Internal Medicine? *New England Journal of Medicine* 317:567-69.

Mechanic, D. 1986. *From Advocacy to Allocation: The Evolving American Health Care System.* New York: Free Press.

Miller, S.J. 1970. *Prescription for Leadership: Training for the Medical Elite.* Chicago: Aldine.

Milman, M. 1977. *The Unkindest Cut: Life in the Backrooms of Medicine.* New York: William Morrow.

Mizrahi, T. 1986. *Getting Rid of Patients: Contradictions in the Socialization of Physicians.* New Brunswick: Rutgers University Press.

Morgan, E. 1980. *The Making of a Woman Surgeon.* New York: G.P. Putnam.

Mullan, F. 1976. *White Coat, Clenched Fist: The Political Education of an American Physician.* New York: Macmillan.

Mumford, E. 1970. *Interns: From Students to Physicians.* Cambridge: Harvard University Press.

Ness, R., C.D. Killian, D.E. Ness, J.B. Frost, and D. McMahon. 1989. Likelihood of Contact with AIDS Patients as a Factor in Medical Students' Residency Selections. *Academic Medicine* 64:588-94.

Nolen, W. 1970. *The Making of a Surgeon.* New York: Random House.

O'Connor, T.W. 1990. Do Patients Have the Right to Infect Their Doctors? *Australia and New Zealand Journal of Surgery* 60:157-62.

Pellegrino, E.D. 1987. Altruism, Self-interest, and Medical Ethics. *Journal of the American Medical Association* 258:1939-40.

Peterson, L.M. 1989. AIDS: The Ethical Dilemma for Surgeons. *Law, Medicine, and Health Care* 17(Summer):139-44.

Ponsford, G. 1987. AIDS in the OR: A Surgeon's View. *Canadian Medical Association Journal* 137:1036-39.

Rabkin, M. 1982. The SAG Index. *New England Journal of Medicine* 307:1350-51.

Reilly, P. 1987. *To Do No Harm: A Journey through Medical School.* Dover, Mass.: Auburn House.

Relman, A.S. 1980. The New Medical-Industrial Complex. *New England Journal of Medicine* 303:963-70.

Rosenberg, J.L., D.P. Jones, L.R. Lipitz, and J.B. Kirsner. 1973. Viral Hepatitis: An Occupational Hazard to Surgeons. *Journal of the American Medical Association* 223:395-400.

Rubin, T.I. 1972. *Emergency Room Diary.* New York: Grosset and Dunlap.

Scully, D. 1980. *Men Who Control Women's Health.* Boston: Houghton Mifflin.

Sharp, S.C. 1988. The Physician's Obligation to Treat AIDS Patients. *Southern Medical Journal* 81:1282–85.

Shem, S. 1978. *The House of God*. New York: Richard Marek.

Shilts, R. 1987. *And the Band Played On*. New York: St. Martins.

Starr, P. 1982. *The Social Transformation of American Medicine*. New York: Basic Books.

Steiner, J.F., L.E. Feinberg, A.M. Kramer, and R.L. Byyny. 1987. Changing Patterns of Disease on an Inpatient Medical Service: 1961–62 to 1981–82. *American Journal of Medicine* 83:331–35.

Stelling, J., and R. Bucher. 1972. Autonomy and Monitoring on Hospital Wards. *Sociological Quarterly* 13:431–47.

Sweeney, III. W. 1973. *Woman's Doctor: A Year in the Life of an Obstetrician-Gynecologist*. New York: Morrow.

Wachter, R.M. 1986. The Impact of the Acquired Immunodeficiency Syndrome on Medical Residency Training. *New England Journal of Medicine* 314:177–80.

X, Dr. 1965. *Intern*. New York: Harper and Row.

Zuger, A. 1987. AIDS on the Wards: A Residency in Medical Ethics. *Hastings Center Report* 17(3):16–20.

Zuger, A., and S.H. Miles. 1987. Physicians, AIDS, and Occupational Risk: Historical Traditions and Ethical Obligations. *Journal of the American Medical Association* 258:1924–28.

Acknowledgments: The listing of the authors reflects the alphabet rather than the efforts of the contributors. This is in every sense an equal collaboration. The authors gratefully acknowledge the contributions of our informants, who must remain nameless. Helpful comments on earlier drafts were made by Robert Arnold and Harold Bershady.

AIDS Volunteering
Links to the Past and Future Prospects

SUZANNE C. OUELLETTE KOBASA

S OON AFTER AIDS WAS FIRST RECOGNIZED IN 1981, concerned lay individuals initiated efforts to deal with the unique crises to which they bore witness. These volunteers came together in associations to do what many others in society were either unwilling or unable to do. They gathered and spread information about the frightening new disease. They raised money to fund much-needed medical research. They cared for those who were suffering, attempting to relieve the horrors caused by both the disease itself and the effects of stigmatization and discrimination. The associations challenged governmental and health authorities to intervene more directly to check the epidemic.

In effect, the work of these early—and subsequent—voluntary associations founded to combat AIDS collectively may come to represent the apotheosis of "the consumer movement." Owing in large part to their efforts, persons with HIV infection are no longer viewed as passive "patients" but rather as "people with AIDS," i.e., as active consumers. The conditions of consumer sovereignty are clearly established and accepted, even if not yet fully met. This outcome can be seen clearly in the effect voluntary associations have had in devising a shared vocabulary about AIDS with the professions, in working jointly to create new knowledge—both social and scientific—and in occupying a preeminent role in defining unmet needs and the conditions under which available services can be made truly accessible to those with HIV infection.

During the past eight years, individual volunteers and voluntary associations have thus played essential roles. Federal agencies, such as the National Institutes of Health and the National Institute of Mental Health, as well as mayoral and gubernatorial offices, have come to invite association representatives to participate in important advisory groups. In New York City, a formal task force on AIDS at the Mayor's Voluntary Action Center includes representatives from 20 community-based organizations and 12 hospital-based volunteer programs; each borough of the city now also has its own volunteer and self-help HIV/AIDS organization. Professional associations influential in American health policy (e.g., Institute of Medicine, National Academy of Sciences 1986) and individual experts (e.g., Fineberg 1988) alike unequivocally describe volunteer community-based organizations as keys to much of the success that society has achieved in its response to AIDS. People who have done AIDS volunteer work (Katoff and Dunne 1988; Lopez and Getzel 1984, 1987) chronicle the unprecedented individual and group needs provoked by AIDS and the successful structures and processes that volunteers have created to meet them. Written by compassionate individuals well experienced in organizational efficiency, these accounts have inspired the replication of volunteer programs both in this country and abroad (Altman 1988; Deucar 1984).

The type, number, and impact of volunteer contributions call for a systematic review that considers not only the effectiveness of AIDS volunteering in the face of the epidemic but also its implications for social and individual life in America. My thesis is that AIDS voluntary activities and associations reveal important facts about how we, as individuals and as a society, respond to crises. These phenomena also corroborate some old ideas about who we are and what we value as Americans. They have to do with notions about the "proper role" of government and the importance of citizens "doing for themselves." AIDS voluntary associations define and press for what government should do; monitor shortfalls of government actions; and provide for needs that are inherently beyond bureaucratic capability. For individuals, participation in AIDS voluntary associations offers an opportunity for empowerment and personal development through social action. Volunteering encourages people to respond successfully to the serious stressors of contemporary life and to see the world as a place in which they can effect important change.

There is good social-science precedent for thinking that one can learn a great deal about individuals and society by looking closely at voluntary associations. Classical nineteenth- and early twentieth-century sociologists studied voluntary associations to understand social change and the redefining of roles and power relationships within society. Alexis de Tocqueville ([1835]1945), for example, viewed voluntary associations as reflective of the essential and distinctive values of a society. A similar notion appears in the study by Robert Bellah and his colleagues (1985) of contemporary American life. They portray voluntary associations as a traditional means by which Americans have sought to understand and express themselves and find significance in public life. Psychologists also have investigated volunteers. M. Brewster Smith (1966) cogently uses the Peace Corps as a context in which to understand "positive mental health" or the more positive aspects of human functioning that are usually left unexplored by psychology. Smith concludes that voluntary organizations are a critical means by which individuals' needs can be effectively integrated with society's requirements.

In what follows, I will use insights from the social sciences to examine some aspects of AIDS volunteering in the United States. The phenomenon has grown to include associations across this country in both large and small cities; the National AIDS Network (NAN) had more than 500 member agencies in 1990. I focus, however, on the oldest and largest AIDS-specific organization, the Gay Men's Health Crisis (GMHC) in New York City. This organization has served and continues to serve as a model for other associations across this country and the world. Understanding GMHC and how it is similar to as well as different from other AIDS efforts is key to grasping the larger phenomenon of AIDS volunteering.

I first describe the essential features of GMHC—how it came to be formed and how it has successfully functioned in society. Second, I will specify the ongoing problems of GMHC and other AIDS voluntary associations that threaten their continued effectiveness; and third, I will speculate on how AIDS voluntary associations might effectively meet these challenges. Tocqueville and David Sills (1968) provide the conceptual framework for the first task. The second integrates their work with contemporary discussions of the achievements and limitations of GMHC and similar AIDS associations, most notably, the critiques of

Peter Arno (1988), Larry Kramer (1987), and Dennis Altman (1988). The final section introduces a more psychological perspective, drawing on work such as that of Smith (1966) and the author's own observations of individuals under stress, to examine more closely what volunteers actually do think, and feel, and to frame speculations on the future of AIDS volunteering.

Tocqueville and the Story of the Gay Men's Health Crisis

Tocqueville's observations of American society date back over a century and a half but they prove remarkably apt for capturing GMHC. Illustrations of his concepts abound in reports of how gay men responded to AIDS by Shilts (1988) and other chroniclers of the epidemic. The framework that Tocqueville offers for the study of voluntary associations usefully distinguishes between how an association is formed and how an association functions.

For this nineteenth-century observer, there are three critical steps in the process by which a collection of people combine to form an association. It begins with people experiencing their inability as isolated individuals to accomplish something that is important to them *and* to oblige existing powers within society to do it for them.

In 1980 gay men began to feel their powerlessness to fend off the seemingly disparate — yet somehow related — array of mysterious illnesses in their midst. Small groups began to come together in writer Larry Kramer's apartment in the summer of 1981 for self-education. They listened attentively to a physician describe a disease spreading like an epidemic among gay men in New York City. He called for help in getting the word out among their friends about its existence and possible links with patterns of sexual behavior and history of venereal disease. A large sum of money ($7,000) was collected that first night in response to the physician's request for funds needed to continue his research on what was then being called "gay cancer" — funds he had been unable to obtain from traditional sources. Five months later, a smaller number of these men met again officially to form an organization to continue the fund raising with a president and board of directors and formal title, the "Gay Men's Health Crisis."

As they went out to do their work — drawing up lists for Mayor Edward I. Koch of what the city needed to be doing in response to the epidemic, detailing gaps and shortfalls in service provision, monitoring and attempting to correct how persons with AIDS (PWAs) were being treated by health care professionals, and providing advice through a hotline and a variety of counseling and direct care services to individuals affected by the disease—GMHC volunteers repeatedly met long-standing prejudices against homosexuals. Individuals with the illness and gay men labeled potential victims of it were suffering social ostracism and the abuse of their basic rights (Lopez and Getzel 1984). In this atmosphere, gay men realized that they would have to continue to turn to each other for help; it would not flow easily from official health providers in society. Even those physicians, both gay and straight, who joined them early on in their struggles felt powerless to get health care institutions to respond appropriately and quickly to the growing crisis.

Tocqueville's second step involves volunteers' recognition of the paradoxes and difficulties inherent in forming associations. Voluntary associations must be large if they are to have clout. But large size prevents volunteers from easily becoming acquainted, understanding each other, fully sharing in a collective agenda and priorities, and establishing fixed regulations—processes that Tocqueville sees as essential to forming an association.

The founding documents in the archives of GMHC make it plain that the first volunteers confronted this issue of size. On the one hand, GMHC scored financial successes with the fund raisers at Paradise Garage in April 1982 and Madison Square Garden in 1983, which drew remarkably large crowds representing a broad-based support from the gay and lesbian community. On the other hand, the majority of people who came to make up the GMHC staff and volunteers were not previously familiar with each other and had little in common other than their mutual concern about the dread new disease. Those gay men who came together to form GMHC as an association were not already part of a single, well-defined, and cohesive social movement. These early GMHC volunteers were not the gay activists of a prior decade; they shared neither ideologies nor opinions about how organizations should be run. Although individual founders, such as Larry Kramer, had been visible and vocal in their struggle to define a political, social, and cultural character for the gay community, the members of this community needed to be organized in a critical new way if their association were to respond effectively to a challenge as formidable as AIDS (cf. Altman 1986).

Conditions for forming such associations were more favorable in San Francisco, the other initial center of the epidemic, than in New York City. San Francisco's gay citizens had in the 1970s achieved a higher degree of social and political cohesion and acceptance, including formal representation in municipal government. The onset of AIDS, however, compelled the gay community there to give priority to AIDS, along with civil rights issues, on their agenda. In contrast, GMHC, as its name makes clear, was a highly specific and ad hoc organization without a historical or parallel political agenda. The group's apparent apolitical nature in serving a nonpolitically defined community of interest undoubtedly made GMHC a less threatening representative to deal with in official quarters.

Tocqueville's ([1835] 1945,114-15) third step, and the one responsible for the success of American associations, involved the "extreme skill with which the inhabitants of the United States succeed in proposing a common object for the exertions of a great many men and inducing them voluntarily to pursue it." Such skill was evident among the founders of GMHC. These men represented a diversified and extensive set of business, corporate, and professional backgrounds. These were successful people who were able to combine their experience to form a voluntary association. They applied what they were practicing in hospital administration, social work, advertising, banking, and other fields to build a successful organizational structure. In addition, a critical few enjoyed substantial financial resources that they were willing to share with the new association to facilitate its solid and visible establishment.

GMHC, over the past eight years, has been able to recruit over 8,000 people to volunteer. Its effectiveness "in proposing a common object" is reflected in the service statistics for the month of August 1989: GMHC volunteers worked with 2,591 clients; answered 5,101 hotline calls; distributed 29,269 pieces of literature; and investigated 210 new complaints against service providers (Gay Men's Health Crisis 1989).

Tocqueville's ideas on how, once established, voluntary associations function also apply to GMHC. Voluntary associations, he postulated, (a) provide services to citizens, (b) define and critique what other parts of society—notably government—should do for those citizens, (c) serve as examples for others in society, and (d) enrich our civilization by attempts "to keep alive and to renew the circulation of opinions and feelings among a great people" ([1835]1945,117).

Volunteers have certainly been essential in providing a full range of services to a growing client base in New York City. To date, GMHC volunteers have worked with over 9,000 clients, serving up to one-third of the people with AIDS living in New York City. Although paid staff at GMHC are involved in the selection, training, supervising, and supporting of the volunteer work, it is the volunteers who actually provide the vast bulk of services.

The active role of associations in large part reflects their expectations of government playing a limited role in confronting social problems. When government in fact is unwilling or unable to do what is needed, voluntary associations step in and take over. GMHC has responded to the failure of existing hospital, welfare, and other social institutions, continually monitoring the workings of these institutions.

Most illness-related volunteer groups act as auxiliaries to established organizations — hospitals, cancer societies, Alzheimer's federations — and further the parent organizations' goals through educational and fundraising missions. GMHC is unusual in its proactive challenge to singular authority and presumed knowledge of professional and governmental agencies about service needs. As it assesses what policies and programs are needed to deal with the epidemic, GMHC rejects the common notion of volunteer as mere auxiliary to established authority. It directly contributes crucial services and demands others, criticizing, for example, the directions of the original HIV presidential commission and the proposals for mandatory testing, name reporting, and contact tracing.

Once citizens have identified each other and formed a strong force, Tocqueville maintains, they can then serve as models for others in society, offering examples and speaking a language to which those outside the organization attend. GMHC has become such a model. In the words of a former executive director, "GMHC is on everyone's list." It now appears to be de rigueur for all levels of government to include a representative of GMHC in any major AIDS-related group that they establish. The media as well seem now naturally to turn to GMHC for its comments and interpretations on AIDS developments, such as in reporting of findings on the effectiveness of AZT administered prior to serious symptom display, and the implications of these results for advising people to take the HIV test.

Finally, according to Tocqueville ([1835]1945,117), voluntary associations provide a setting in which "[f]eelings and opinions are recruited, the heart is enlarged, and the human mind is developed." To leave the job of enriching civilization to government would result inevitably in either tyranny or torpor. The founders and long-term leaders of GMHC evinced this view. In his first major address as the first president of the GMHC board of directors, Paul Popham expressed the power he felt in men having come together and the inspiring message that they would be able to communicate to themselves as well as others:

> It may be that equal measure of fear and hope has brought us together, but the great thing is, we *are* together. . . . We've got to fight back. . . . We've got to show each other and the unfriendly world that we've got more than looks, brains, talent, and money. We've got guts too, plus an awful lot of heart (Shilts 1988, 139).

Lopez and Getzel (1987, 53) refer to the lessons about human compassion they find in the voluntary response to AIDS:

> We must set in place a skilled, humane network of concerned and trained human-service professionals and volunteers as our response to the AIDS epidemic. In so doing, we not only help persons with AIDS in a significant way until a definite medical break-through occurs, but we preserve our collective humanity and social solidarity against the impulse of indifference and cruelty.

Sills and Analysis of GMHC

One hundred and thirty-three years later, David Sills (1968) elaborated on Tocqueville's basic vision, bringing modern sociological and political science critiques of organizational function to bear on the role of voluntary associations. Sills classifies voluntary associations in several ways. Most useful for our purposes are his categories for distinguishing between organizations in terms of what they do and how they are organized.

GMHC and most other AIDS organizations are volunteer health agencies with the primary function of providing *direct services* to persons affected by illness. GMHC's "buddies" provide practical physical and emotional support on a day-to-day basis, while some of its other volunteers provide financial and legal advice on the many complicated problems accompanying AIDS. AIDS organizations also carry out other essential functions. These include *fund raising*, geared to the financial support of AIDS research as well as care-related programs; *education and reduction of AIDS risk*, directed to the population at large, particular groups of individuals thought to be at especially high risk, and medical and mental health professionals responsible for the care of PWAs; *advocacy*, aimed at giving voice to those with HIV illness and mediating between PWAs and several major social institutions including governmental, medical, and scientific organizations; and *policy*, entailing the lobbying of political authorities at local, state, and national levels to initiate as well as improve their responses to AIDS, and working with the media to heighten their sensitivity and responsible reporting on AIDS issues.

In categorizing current AIDS voluntary efforts, many organizations (especially smaller ones) function as single-purpose associations. The People With AIDS Coalition, for example, focuses largely on advocacy. The Community Research Initiative stresses reduction of AIDS risk through its mounting of alternative and efficient forms of drug testing. As for direct service organizations, God's Love We Deliver brings cooked meals to the homes of PWAs, Pet Owners With AIDS Resource Services (POWARS) organizes walks for PWAs' pets, and the Manhattan Plaza AIDS Project (in what can be one of the most isolating and anomie-provoking cities in the world) organizes neighbors within a high-rise apartment complex to help care for each other. GMHC and other large AIDS organizations must be recognized, however, as unusual among voluntary health associations in carrying out all these various functions simultaneously.

Relevant to an understanding of how AIDS associations are organized, Sills distinguishes two basic sorts of associations: "formal-organization-like associations" and "social-movement-like associations." The former, exemplified by organizations like the American Cancer Society and the American Red Cross, are aimed at gradual and conventionally accepted improvement of the social order, and volunteers participate with low emotional commitment. Typically, the organizational structure is formalized and fixed. The latter may span groups as different as Planned Parenthood and World Zionist Congress, whose radical and ideological programs are likely to be at some variance with the status quo, and whose volunteers are emotionally involved. Their organizational structure is more informal and fluid.

Using this classificatory scheme, GMHC as an association faces potential dissonance: its programs and volunteer spirit mark it as one sort of association and its structure as another. When considered in the broad context of all American voluntary associations, GMHC clearly has to be placed within the social-movement-like half of the world. Its formal mission contains the goals of advocacy and policy change. Its volunteer participants typically bring high levels of emotional commitment to their work. This is particularly true for those who are motivated to volunteer as a way of either coping with losses they have personally experienced, or expressing the anger they feel at society at large for failing to respond to the epidemic without discrimination against and stigmatization of PWAs.

Viewed in the light of its own history, however, the current structure of GMHC reflects some of the characteristics of a formal-organization-like association. Increasing institutionalization and formalization have accompanied the growth of GMHC, whose staff payroll totals 140 people. The immediate past executive director gained extensive managerial training in the corporate world. While there has been a rise in the numbers of clients and volunteers, expansion of formal structures and bureaucratic processes has taken place. In 1984, Lopez and Getzel succinctly described the service model that GMHC created simply by telling the story of an individual PWA and the individual volunteers working with him. Four years later, Katoff and Dunne (1988) provided an update on the model by listing and describing the eight formal components that make up client services, reviewing such features as how information is recorded and transferred from department to department and the supervisory structures in which volunteers participate. The volunteer is no longer expected to have direct contact with staff at GMHC but rather to communicate through his or her team leader with those running the association. Sills's perspective makes plain the tension between increasing institutionalization at GMHC and preservation of the organization's social-movement character.

Sills also specifies mechanisms through which an association comes to manifest excessive institutionalization. The two most important ones involve the "iron law of oligarchy" and "goal displacement." With regard to the former, Sills quotes Michels ([1911]1959) to describe how a fully democratic system within a voluntary association can be quickly replaced by an oligarchic form in which a small elite holding leadership positions solely make decisions. As for his second mechanism, goal displacement, the association's activities come to be centered around the proper functioning of organizational structures and processes *rather than* the reaching of goals for which the association was founded. Both of these mechanisms according to Sills lead to an organizational climate in which current volunteers feel that they no longer have any say in shaping the association's work and potential volunteers or recruits complain that they do not clearly see the mission of the association.

Another way of understanding the institutional tensions GMHC currently confronts is to contrast it with the more recently formed AIDS Coalition to Unleash Power (ACT UP); the popular media often pair the two organizations. ACT UP has succeeded in avoiding the bureaucratic conflicts troubling GMHC by, in the words of one of its prominent participants, "not being a social movement *organization*, but being a social movement." A new member of ACT UP tellingly observes that: "People at GMHC are volunteers — maybe even some of those thousand points of light — people at ACT UP are activists and too angry simply to sit down with George Bush." At its founding, members of ACT UP recognized the shortcomings of institutional authority as necessary consequences of structural deficiencies in official agencies and sought not accommodation — of which it accused GMHC in harsh terms — but challenge and confrontation as its initial and necessary strategies.

ACT UP's tactics, moreover, have gained wide attention for the challenges of AIDS that society has yet to meet through public demonstrations and a repertoire of activities reminiscent of the late 1960s and 1970s. These tactics include street-theater presentations and "Zaps" (acts of civil disobedience designed to focus greater public and government attention on the epidemic). Through these measures, it has avoided the development of a small controlling elite and enabled the majority of its members to feel that they define the agenda of the group.

This is not to say, however, that ACT UP has not had to struggle to avoid its own brand of institutionalization. In a recent article in the *Village Voice*, Minkowitz (1990) recounts how a small group of ACT UP members, including Larry Kramer, brought before the group a proposal to create an "administrative committee" capable of making decisions without approval from the floor. When subjected to ACT UP's rigorously democratic process (which allows all members to vote on organizational actions), the proposal's supporter was elected as the new ACT UP administrator only after lengthy and bitter debate. ACT UP is becoming subject to internal dissonance in matters such as renewal of old commitments versus constantly evolving agendas; seeking parity among the many and varied claimants for action, including women and minority-group members; and addressing tensions between advocating different national strategies for meeting the costs of health care.

Ongoing Problems of AIDS Voluntary Associations: Contemporary Critiques

Much of what has been written about AIDS voluntary associations has been congratulatory. The most articulate contemporary commentators, however, document limitations as well as achievements of organizations like GMHC. Arno (1986, 1988), for example, has done formal studies revealing the positive economic impact of AIDS volunteering. Through activities like broad-based case management that provide continuity of care to PWAs and facilitate effective care-giving by family and friends as well as health care personnel, AIDS volunteering helps PWAs remain outside of a hospital or reduce length of stay in a hospital. Arno's data show that case-management efforts are efficient, placing little drain on the larger society. Most of GMHC's work is done by unpaid volunteers and only a small part of its revenue comes from government sources. At the end of 1987, the ratio of unpaid to paid staff hours at GMHC was ten times higher than the average ratio at other service agencies in the city, despite a doubling of paid staff in that year. In that same year, GMHC drew 70 percent of its revenues from private donations.

Arno also, however, details some significant problems. He questions whether society as a whole may have come to rely too much and too exclusively on the contributions of volunteers. The current volunteer force may not be able to meet the needs of the new populations affected by AIDS. Many of the volunteers are gay men, he notes, a pool already depleted either by the illness itself or by commitments to other AIDS-related work. Many voluntary associations are unfamiliar with the particular needs of the ethnic minority communities that are now experiencing the most significant rise in AIDS cases. Others that are familiar may be without sufficient resources to address the numerous crises that accompany AIDS as it expands among groups already beset by poverty, high crime rates, drug abuse, and racial discrimination.

Arno's views are reinforced and elaborated by Larry Kramer (1985, 1987). Using a variety of settings — the stage, newspaper columns, and public demonstrations — Kramer, a disaffected founder of GMHC who has become a major figure in ACT UP, acidly accuses voluntary associations like GMHC and their leaders of being so politically timid and preoccupied with preservation of their own status that they have allowed local, state, and federal government to renege on their promises to do something about AIDS.

Kramer criticizes two facets of GMHC's organizational commitment to delivering services to PWAs. Offering care takes association resources and volunteers' energies away from activism and the formulation of a politically viable radical alternative to the government's position on AIDS, and it relieves government of service responsibilities and obligations. Kramer's point is that we would be facing a less bleak future if government had funded massive research and initiated reforms in the organization, delivery, and financing of the entire health care system.

Altman (1986, 1988), a political scientist studying voluntary associations within the history of gay organizations and gay politics, is also critical. He concludes that, on the one hand, the forming of communal organizations to deal with the epidemic has strengthened the idea of a gay community. For through voluntary association, gay men have increased their involvement in the political process. On the other hand, it has brought new tensions to the gay community. For example, the links between AIDS voluntary associations and various government agencies increase the gay community's dependence on government. The emergence of AIDS experts, not necessarily representative of the gay community in terms of class, race, and age, contributes to strain. These experts have strong professional credentials and are practiced at dealing with bureaucracies, but they may fail to speak for the entire community.

GMHC and other AIDS voluntary associations are at a critical juncture in society's attempts to cope with AIDS. They have come a long way in refining their objectives, but these very successes are a source of tension. According to Tocqueville, "If men are to remain civilized or to become so, the art of associating together must grow and improve" ([1835]1945,118). This art will include both the founding of new voluntary associations and the joining of established and new organizations to respond to the continuing epidemic. One promising example of the latter is the recent joint sponsorship by GMHC and Harlem Hospital of a program addressed to the special education and treatment needs of people of color. GMHC and other organizations with a gay constituency have also joined in cooperative initiatives for PWAs with a variety of minority and mainstream service sponsors and providers, such as the Association for Drug Abuse Prevention and Treatment (ADAPT), Federation of Protestant Welfare Agencies, Jewish Board of Family Services, Minority Task Force on AIDS, Partnership for the Homeless, and Retired Senior Volunteer Program.

Another focus of future volunteering will be the reassessment and redefinition of the roles played by each AIDS organization. GMHC and ACT UP, for example, partly reversed "normative" roles at the recent Sixth International AIDS Conference held in San Francisco. Typically criticized by radical factions for being too willing to sit down and talk with the authorities, GMHC chose to boycott the meetings, protesting the government's immigration policies concerning HIV-positive people. ACT UP, the organization that usually shuns collaborative ventures with officials, played an important role in the meetings' deliberations and was joined in particular protests by organizers of the conference. In other demonstrations, however, ACT UP resumed its antiestablishment position. It remains to be seen how and how often internal politics in each organization and external events might impel the two to take unexpected stances on other issues.

Meeting the Challenges of AIDS Volunteering

In speculating on the future of AIDS voluntary associations, we must know more about the psychology of the AIDS volunteer—the individuals who maintain and shape the nature and function of the association. We understand little about the intrapersonal or interpersonal factors that influence initial decisions to volunteer at all, or to choose among such varied opportunities as those offered by ACT UP or GMHC. Such factors are the subject of my current research. How do AIDS volunteers confront all of the various causes of stress that they encounter in their work without becoming debilitated or suffering "burnout"? How do they cope with or avoid emotional exhaustion, lack of sense of accomplishment, and cynical detachment from the clients or patients involved? Drawing on the extensive general literature on stress and its impact on persons' physical and psychological well-being, I have hypothesized in earlier articles that the impact of stressful work depends on the degree of "personality hardiness"—the individual's orientation toward commitment, control, and challenge—brought to the stressful situation (e.g., Kobasa 1982). The stronger the hardiness, that is, the greater the sense of commitment, ability to feel in control, and willingness to confront change, the less the likelihood of burnout.

Observations of volunteering activity offer general support for this hypothesis. The founder-volunteers who shaped the rapid growth, relative stability, organizational development, and fund-raising success of GMHC, for example, appear to have been a hardy group. They knew the horror of the epidemic, yet they felt that there was something they could do to determine the course of events; they were active individuals with many commitments in their personal and working lives; and they were certainly willing to confront uncertainty—viewing the epidemic as a challenge and not a mere threat. Interviews with current as well as former volunteers suggest, moreover, that their sense of political commitment, control, and challenge was developed through participation in the association, and some have found critical new meaning for themselves over the course of their work.

This emergent sense of empowerment developed with experience and competence. Many AIDS volunteers unexpectedly found themselves able to do things beyond the realm of prior experience or expertise. Some went beyond finding satisfaction in assisting PWAs manage domestic tasks through one-on-one encounters to fulfillment in participating in public events designed to engender social change.

The structure and functions of GMHC offer individuals opportunities to develop competence. GMHC's policy-defining and government-monitoring functions provide new roles for volunteers. The success and status that GMHC has earned as an association facilitate volunteers' ability to feel committed and involved in their work. People surveyed talk about how volunteering has allowed them to find a new sense of meaning or purpose (also cf. Kobasa and Maddi 1983, for discussion of the contexts in which this purposive sense may arise). Several, whose paid jobs also involve human service work (nurses, social workers, physicians, psychotherapists) poignantly describe how volunteering has enabled them to find that intimacy with others that had initially motivated their careers. Some of the most satisfied volunteers are those who encountered new cultures, new values, and new ways of relating to others in their fulfillment of their volunteer role. From this perspective, most critical to the future success of GMHC and other voluntary associations is their continued ability to provide such opportunities to individual volunteers. Recognition of their role in fostering empowerment can counterbalance stress and burnout.

The response to AIDS (like that of interest groups focused on all sides of the abortion questions, or on environmental issues) suggest an increasing trend of citizens taking issues of governance into their own hands—through voluntary associations, if not through direct participation in electoral processes. This chapter has tried to elucidate some of the key challenges to these associations. Citizens' movements so admiringly noted by Tocqueville more than 150 years ago remain a force for satisfaction, and possible progress and enlightenment, in American cultural life.

References

Altman, D. 1986. *AIDS in the Mind of America*. Garden City, N.Y.: Anchor Press/Doubleday.

———. 1988. Legitimation through Disaster: AIDS and the Gay Movement. In *AIDS: The Burdens of History*, ed. E. Fee and D.M. Fox, 301–15. Berkeley: University of California Press.

Arno, P.S. 1986. The Nonprofit Sector's Response to the AIDS Epidemic: Community-based Services in San Francisco. *American Journal of Public Health* 76:1325–30.

———. 1988. The Future of Voluntarism and the AIDS Epidemic. In *The AIDS Patient: An Action Agenda*, ed. D. Rogers and E. Ginzberg, 56–70. Boulder: Westview.

Bellah, R.N., R. Madsen, S.M. Sullivan, A. Swidler, and S.M. Tipton. 1985. *Habits of the Heart: Individualism and Commitment in American Life*. New York: Harper and Row.

Deucar, N. 1984. AIDS in New York City with Particular Reference to the Psycho-social Aspects. *British Journal of Psychiatry* 145:612–19.

Fineberg, H.V. 1988. The Social Dimensions of AIDS. *Scientific American* 259:110–20.

Gay Men's Health Crisis. 1989. Vital Statistics. *The Volunteer* 6:11.

Hollander, G. 1988. *Voluntary Management: Development and Maintenance of Volunteer Programs in AIDS Service Organizations*. Washington: National AIDS Network.

Institute of Medicine, National Academy of Sciences. 1986. *Confronting AIDS*. Washington: National Academy Press.

Katoff, L., and R. Dunne. 1988. Supporting People with AIDS: The Gay Men's Health Crisis Model. *Journal of Palliative Care* 4:88–95.

Kobasa, S.C. 1982. The Personality and Social Psychology of Stress and Health. In *Social Psychology of Health and Illness*, ed. G. Sanders and J. Suls, 3–22, Hillsdale, N.J.: Erlbaum.

Kobasa, S.C., and S. Maddi. 1983. Existential Personality Theory. In *Personality Theories, Research, and Assessment*, ed. R.J. Corsini and A.J. Marsella, 399–446. Itasca, Ill.: F.E. Peacock.

Kramer, L. 1985. *The Normal Heart*. New York: New American Library.

————. 1987. Open letter. *New York Native* 197 (January 26): 1, 12.

Lopez, D.J. and G.S. Getzel. 1984. Helping Gay AIDS Patients in Crisis. *Social Casework* 65:387–94.

————. 1987. Strategies for Volunteers Caring for Persons with AIDS. *Social Casework* 68:47–53.

Michels, R. [1911]1959. *Political Parties: A Sociological Study of the Oligarchical Tendencies of Modern Democracy*. New York: Dover.

Minkowitz, D. 1990. ACT UP at a Crossroads. *Village Voice* (June 5):19–22.

Quimby, E., and S.R. Friedman. 1989. Dynamics of Black Mobilization against AIDS in New York City. *Social Problems* 36:403–15.

Shilts, R. 1988. *And the Band Played on: Politics, People, and the AIDS Epidemic*. New York: Penguin Books.

Sills, D.L. 1968. Voluntary Associations. In the *International Encyclopaedia of the Social Sciences*, 357–78. New York: Macmillan.

Smith, M.B. 1966. Explorations in Competence: A Study of Peace Corps Volunteers in Ghana. *American Psychologist* 21:555–66.

Tocqueville, A. de. [1835]1945. *Democracy in America*. New York: Vintage.

Part IV.

Rights and Reciprocities

AIDS and the Future of
Reproductive Freedom

RONALD BAYER

LIBERAL INDIVIDUALISM HAS REPRESENTED A powerful liberating ideological challenge to both the legal moralism that sought to enforce conventional values by state power and the intrusive and restrictive claims of social orthodoxy. The defense of privacy, so central in that confrontation, has defined realms of social life to be protected from coercion and pressure. No reading of the transformations of the past three decades could fail to recognize the achievements of the liberal challenge (Karst 1980). Certainly, the profound, even if fragile, alteration of the moral and legal standards surrounding sexuality and procreation attest to the stunning victory of those who sought to free individuals from intrusive social and public policies. Now that abortion rights, first secured by the 1973 Supreme Court decision in *Roe v. Wade*, have become so vulnerable to the political currents crystalized by the Court in its 1989 *Webster* ruling, the achievements of the liberal ascendency during this era seem all the more striking.

AIDS has represented a challenge to the central impulse of liberal individualism, forcing into the social realm matters that had come to be viewed as of no legitimate public concern; it has revealed the limits of the ideology that had provided the wellspring of cultural and political reform. Pediatric AIDS has contributed yet one more element to the broad encounter with the liberal commitment to the sanctity of reproductive choice, encumbered neither by governmental restrictions nor social pressures. How will the threat of a maternally transmitted lethal infection affect the tolerance for an ethos that has proclaimed the utter privacy of each woman's reproductive decision? Will the grim reality of pediatric AIDS generate pressures for social interventions that would shape, direct, constrain, limit, or control those decisions in ways that might contradict the pronatalist demands of the movement that seeks to restrict severely or eliminate the right to abortion? Much will depend upon how many babies are born infected with HIV and die. Much more will depend on the social perceptions provoked by those numbers.

As of March 1989 about 1,500 cases of AIDS in children below the age of 13 had been reported to the Centers for Disease Control (1989). In approximately 1,200 cases, just over 400 in the last year alone, HIV infection had been vertically transmitted—from mother to fetus; the remaining cases have been linked to blood transfusions or the use of clotting factor in hemophiliacs. With the securing of the safety of the blood supply it is a certainty that virtually all new cases of HIV infection in infants will be the consequence of maternal infection.

Without satisfactory national seroprevalence studies of women of childbearing age and of adolescent girls, some of whom will become pregnant, there is no very good way of estimating the number of infected babies that may be born, nor of projecting the number of pediatric cases of AIDS. The frequency with which infected women transmit infection to their fetuses also remains uncertain, the most commonly suggested range being between 25 and 50 percent. Finally, much will depend upon the extent to which infected women continue to become pregnant and carry their pregnancies to term. Here too, the data are only preliminary. A Brooklyn hospital found no difference between the reproductive decisions of infected and uninfected women (Sunderland et al. 1988). A study conducted at a Bronx methadone maintenance program corroborated those findings. More than 20 percent of both infected and uninfected women had become pregnant during the course of a two-year period. More than 25 percent of those same women became pregnant a second time (Selwyn et al. 1989).

Even more so than is the case with HIV infection in adults, the burden of pediatric AIDS has been geographically concentrated, mimicking the epidemiology of drug addiction. New York, New Jersey, Florida, Texas, California, and Puerto Rico will continue to be the centers of vertical HIV transmission. And even in those regions the prevalence of pediatric HIV disease will be concentrated in particular communities. In New York City, where 1.25 percent of women of childbearing age are infected, hospitals serving neighborhoods with high levels of intravenous drug use have reported rates of infection as high as 4 percent (Novick et al. 1989). At one Newark, New Jersey, hospital the rate was 5 percent (Tom Denney, personal communication).

In sum, although the precise dimensions of the potential problem of pediatric AIDS remain uncertain, it is clear that the number of cases will continue to rise over the next years. The cost in both social and medical resources that will be required to care for such children and the toll in human suffering will not be negligible. An editorial in the *Journal of the American Medical Association* could thus declare: "The contribution of the [progeny of HIV-infected women] to infant mortality in the nation's inner cities will soon dwarf that of other congenital infections such as cytomegalovirus, herpes and syphilis" (Landesman, Willoughby, and Minkoff 1989, 1326).

Just as the threat of transfusion-associated cases of AIDS aroused the deepest of social fears, the specter of maternally transmitted HIV infection has touched the deepest emotions. During the past nine years we have become all too familiar with the capacity of American society — and of other societies as well — to distinguish between the "innocent" victims of the epidemic and those who, however unwittingly, have been implicated in their own unfortunate state. Unable to protect themselves from the decisions of their mothers, HIV-infected babies provide the paradigmatic case of past and future undeserved suffering. But even for those who have rejected as morally irrelevant, and socially divisive, the question of how individuals have become infected and the distinctions between individuals who had become infected before the first cases of AIDS were recognized and those whose behaviors exposed them to risk after much was known about the possibilities of self-protection, the plight of children born to disease and early death continues to be especially poignant, warranting a special urgency.

Like infants suffering the consequences of fetal alcohol syndrome and drug withdrawal, babies with AIDS — the "littlest victims" — provoke the demand for preventive intervention. Here, the reformist zeal that so frequently has attended efforts to save children from their parents' misdeeds may merge with the eugenic tradition of challenging the absolute right of parents to bear children at high risk for congenital disorders, since only a decision not to bear children can prevent the birth of infected infants to infected mothers. It is the specter of such reformist zeal and the legacy of eugenics that haunt the discussion of how to achieve the otherwise unassailable goal of preventing the birth of babies who will die of AIDS.

That the women who are most at risk for bearing infected children are poor, black, and Hispanic, and most often intravenous drug users or their sexual partners, heightens the sense of disquiet about the prospect of a repressive turn in public policy (Centers for Disease Control 1989). How would infected women be identified? What efforts would be made to discourage them from becoming pregnant? How directive and how aggressive would the counseling of such a woman be? What would be the response to those who did become pregnant? Given the increasingly restrictive social regime surrounding abortion, what measures beyond counseling might be employed to prevent the birth of infected infants? The disquiet provoked by concerns about the course of AIDS-related policy has been amplified by the broader challenge to the reproductive freedom of women. Might efforts to limit the toll of pediatric AIDS not only draw upon the movement to restrict the hard-won victories of the 1960s and 1970s but further erode reproductive rights as well? Might such efforts not only draw upon a tradition of subtle eugenic practices but foster the revival of an explicit eugenic ideology?

The most apocalyptic visions of what measures might be taken to control the spread of AIDS involve the wholesale abrogation of the privacy and reproductive freedom of all HIV-infected women, as well as those considered at high risk for infection. Writing in the *Journal of the American Medical Association*, Robert Edelman of the National Institute of Allergy and Infectious Diseases and Harry Haverkos of the National Institute on Drug Abuse argued that the existence of heterosexual transmission of HIV infection in the United States would compel society to confront the question of the "suitability of infected individuals for marriage and natural parenthood" (Edelman and Haverkos 1989). The logic of seeking to enforce standards of "suitability" for procreation would of necessity lead to mandatory and repeated testing of all women of reproductive age, criminalized childbirth, coerced abortion, or compulsory sterilization. Although opposed to such repressive interventions, Edelman and Haverkos nevertheless warn that the demand for effective prophylaxis might well create a climate within which coercion would become tolerable: "We can predict that as the pandemic widens and deepens in our society, increasingly powerful voices will be heard calling for such state imposed restrictions."

The possibility of such massive coercion—despite the array of ethical, legal, constitutional, political, and logistical objections that would be provoked—has also been noted by Norman Fost, chair of the bioethics committee of the American Academy of Pediatrics. Locating the problem of HIV infection in both historical and contemporary sociopolitical contexts, he has sounded an alarm. More than 100,000 retarded women were sterilized in the period between 1920 and 1973 on the assumption that they could transmit their condition to their children. Both the prospect of the social burden of having to support an ever-increasing population of "incompetents" and the specter that they would in turn bear retarded children provided the eugenic basis for such interventions. "If the country could get behind that it surely could get behind sterilizing women to prevent a much more serious problem." The vulnerability of women's reproductive freedom, given the current political climate, he asserted, increased the likelihood of a repressive turn in public policy. "There is," Fost stated, "a very powerful legal trend for intrusion on women for social reasons" (Abraham 1988).

Whether such drastic measures on so wide a scale will be provoked by the AIDS epidemic in the next years cannot be predicted. In the first years of the epidemic, gay men were able to articulate forcefully the importance of preserving the values of privacy in the face of a lethal viral challenge, and public health officials in alliance with liberal political leaders came to recognize that reliance on repressive measures could well subvert the prospects of prevention. The result was a voluntarist political culture that shaped the main currents of AIDS policy (Bayer 1989). Much will depend on the extent to which that culture will survive the epidemic's next years in which hundreds of thousands of already infected persons will become profoundly and fatally ill. But in the absence of a dramatic erosion of the basic premises of voluntarism it is unlikely that harsh and repressive reproductive policies will emerge. More likely, there will be aggressive campaigns to dissuade infected women from bearing children. Ironically, the prospects for avoiding coercive policies may, at least in part, depend on the success of such persuasive interventions.

But even such measures will require a confrontation with the broadly shared perspective that has evolved over the past two decades on matters of reproductive choice. Because of the chronic nature of HIV infection, recommendations to women about their childbearing decisions will entail efforts to shape their entire reproductive lives. In that way, and because of the uncertainty of maternal transmission, the quandaries raised by HIV infection are much more like those posed by the risks of transmitting genetic disorders than by acute conditions. It was precisely with regard to the questions of public policy and clinical practice in the face of the risks of genetic disorders that the importance of preserving the right of women to make reproductive decisions had taken hold, unencumbered by political, professional, or social pressures. Shaped by the professional ethos of genetic counseling, medical ethics, and feminist thought, the ideology of nondirective counseling achieved hegemony, reflecting a singular commitment to liberal individualism. AIDS will surely challenge that ideology.

Genetic Counseling and Reproductive Choice

It was against the legacy of eugenics that the very term genetic counseling was coined in the post-World War II years. Unlike the eugenics movement—which had been driven by class, nativist, and racist concerns for the protection of the genetic stock (Ludmerer 1972; Kevles 1985)—the new practice was to be a "type of social work entirely for the benefit of the whole family without direct concern for its effect upon the state or politics" (Reed 1974, 336). Since neither the well-being of the community nor that of future generations was pertinent to the counselor's work, the professional task was to assist individuals confronted with the prospect of bearing children with genetic disorders to select "the course of action which seems appropriate to them in view of their risks and their family goals and to act in accordance with that decision" (Fraser 1974). In the years before the technology of prenatal diagnoses became available and in the era before *Roe v. Wade* had recognized the right of a woman to terminate her pregnancy, the purview of genetic counseling was of necessity largely restricted to preconceptual decisions. It was the scientific advance represented by amniocentesis and political change represented by the Supreme Court's 1973 abortion decision that made possible the extension of the scope of genetic counseling to the full range of reproductive decisions.

Remarkably, the commitment to nondirective counseling, so discordant with the traditions of clinical medicine, attained hegemonic status not only in the United States but also abroad. The Expert Committee on Human Genetics of the World Health Organization (1968) and the National Academy of Sciences (1975) both warned against eugenic goals and underscored the importance of a counseling process that permitted individuals to make choices free of pressure. Surveys of counselor attitudes both in the United States (Sorenson, Swazey, and Scotch 1981, 44) and abroad (Wertz and Fletcher 1988) demonstrated how profoundly the ideology of nondirective counseling had shaped professional attitudes. In one widely cited survey of American counselors, only 13 percent of those studied believed it appropriate to "advise patients about what to do." Just 20 percent considered it appropriate to help shape patients' decisions by informing them about what they themselves might do in similar situations (Sorenson, Swazey, and Scotch 1981, 44).

Despite the fact that evaluations of genetic counseling frequently revealed a commitment to reducing the fertility of those at risk for bearing children with genetic disorders (Bird 1985; Reed 1980), the recognition of the inevitable intrusion, however subtle, of personal values as counselors seek to guide their clients (Katz Rothman 1986; Rapp 1988), and the resurgent interest in eugenic goals in the face of enhanced diagnostic capabilities (Nelkin and Tancredi 1989; Perry 1981), the ethos of nondirective counseling has retained its dominance both as a professional ideology and as a guiding principle for public agencies.

Bioethics, Autonomy, and
Reproductive Freedom

Paralleling the concerns of genetic counselors about professional coercion were those of the intellectuals who forged the discipline of bioethics. Emerging out of the turbulence of the 1960s and marked by the imprint of liberal individualism, the new field sought to provide a moral foundation for the enhanced power of patients. Against medical paternalism the antidote was autonomy. It is not surprising that the rapid developments in genetics—part of the "biological revolution"—drew the interest of bioethics, since such advances opened the prospect of medicalized social control. Just three years after its founding, the

Hastings Center (Institute of Society, Ethics, and the Life Sciences) produced ethical guidelines on genetic counseling that were antagonistic to both legal coercion and professional practices that might subvert the capacity of individuals to choose for themselves the appropriate reproductive course. Published in the *New England Journal of Medicine* and endorsed by virtually every figure identified with the creation of contemporary bioethics, these recommendations represented a seminal element in the emerging public consensus on genetic counseling (Institute of Society, Ethics, and the Life Sciences 1972).

The centrality of individual choice as a moral norm for genetic counseling, though consonant with the main currents of bioethics, has not gone unchallenged. From the beginning there were those who believed that the obligation to prevent harm required reproductive restraint on the part of individuals at high risk for bearing children who would suffer. At a minimum, such restraint would have made the use of contraceptive methods morally imperative (Callahan 1979). At its most extreme this perspective not only rejected the nondirective approach to counseling but urged legal restraints on those who might bear "defective" children (Shaw 1984). Drawing on the thoroughgoing utilitarianism that often set him at odds with the dominant trends in bioethics, Joseph Fletcher (1980, 132) argued:

> There are more Typhoid Marys carrying genetic diseases than infectious disease. If infectious diseases are sometimes grave enough to justify both ethical and legal restrictions on carriers why not some genetic diseases too? . . . We ought in conscience to have a humane minimum standard of reproduction, not blindly accept the outcome of every conception.

How marginal such views remained was underscored by the 1982 report on genetic screening by the President's Commission on Ethical Problems in Medicine and Biomedical and Behavioral Research (1982). Like the work of the Hastings Center conducted a decade earlier, the commission report was marked by liberal individualism's anticoercive, antipaternalistic orientation. Genetic screening and counseling, the report asserted, could serve to enhance human options but could, like other advances in medicine, deprive individuals of the capacity for self-determination. Autonomy could be threatened not only by governmental restrictions but by professional dominance. Both, in turn, would subvert the possibility of truly free choice. "Someone who feels compelled to undergo screening or to make a particular reproductive choice at the urging of health care professionals or others as a result of implicit social pressures is deprived of the choice-enhancing benefits of the new advances."

Feminism and Procreative Rights

The contemporary feminist movement has contributed an explicitly political dimension to the professional and philosophical foundations of nondirective counseling. Central to feminism has been the assertion that women be permitted to determine their own reproductive lives, the demand for access to birth control and abortion services, the insistence that women be free of threats to the right to bear children, and, increasingly, that they be free to control the method, circumstances, and timing of the exercise of that right (Katz Rothman 1986; Ruzek 1978). "The notion of choice has served as an ideological cornerstone of the political program of the movement for reproductive rights and women's health" (Wikler 1986, 1049). Despite its divergent ideological roots and despite its concern with the collective experience and needs of women, the mainstream of American feminism has thus been profoundly influenced by the central tenets of liberal individualism.

The feminist perspective of genetic screening and counseling must be seen within this context. On the one hand, the information provided by such services has been viewed as extending the opportunity of women to make informed choices about whether to conceive and carry pregnancies to term. On the other hand, genetic diagnosis has been feared because of the dangerous prospect of the emergence of standards of "appropriate" reproductive decisions (Katz Rothman 1986, 23). "It is not acceptable that the understandable desire of many women to have as healthy a baby as possible would become a duty aimed at the welfare of the gene pool" (Stanworth 1987, 31). Barbara Katz Rothman's (1986) widely read *Tentative Pregnancy* represents an impassioned analysis of prenatal diagnosis which warns that the new reproductive technologies might ironically constrain choice by expanding the possibility for choice. Are we, she asks, losing the right not to choose?

Because of the historically rooted experience of women who have been the subjects of restrictive reproductive policy and professional practices, feminist discussion of genetic counseling has often centered on the important, but difficult to detail, disjunction between the reality and the official ethos of nondirective clinical behavior (Rose 1987). Alert to the empirical research that has demonstrated the subtly directive content of counseling that guides choices despite the claim to neutrality, feminists have been sharply critical of the "unbalanced" and distorting information which limits the options available to women. Thus, they have argued, for example, that the emphasis within counseling upon the burdens of bearing a child with some congenital defect denies prospective parents the opportunity to make reproductive choices in the light of the possibility that such a child could be a source of fulfillment (Hubbard 1988).

Given this perspective, it is not surprising that feminists have viewed substantive and public discussions of how women should exercise their reproductive options as threatening an erosion of always precarious reproductive freedoms. But despite such anxiety, current feminist literature has been compelled to address these matters. Radical theoreticians like Rosalind Petchesky (1984, 6), in search of a feminist/socialist ethic, have attempted to transcend the limits of individualism in order to confront "moral questions about when, under what conditions and for what purposes reproductive decisions should be made." Those allied to the disability rights movement, like Adrienne Asch (1989), have been troubled by the assumption that efforts to preclude the birth of less than perfect children are beyond moral scrutiny. And those alert to the potentially antifeminist implications of some reproductive choices that women, influenced by the broader culture, might make — aborting female fetuses because of a preference for male children (Hoskins and Holmes 1984) or agreeing to enter into maternal surrogacy agreements — have even begun to entertain the question of whether the absolutist defense of choice is still tenable (Wikler 1986). But with some few exceptions feminist writers still embrace, if only for strategic reasons, unrestricted reproductive decision making. Asch (1989, 82) has written, "I may deplore what some women do, but I am not yet prepared to take away their rights of self-determination." It is this commitment to self-determination that has defined the enduring feminist perspective on nondirective reproductive counseling.

It is against this rich, professionally and politically rooted, ideology of privacy in reproductive decision making that the response to the threat of vertical HIV transmission must be viewed. Officials involved with AIDS prevention activities were often very distant from the concerns of those who had forged this ideological perspective. At times they seemed utterly uncomprehending of the sensitivities surrounding reproductive choice, especially those rooted in the fears of poor black and Hispanic women whose awareness of past policies of coercive sterilization would inevitably produce resistance to any form of directive fertility control. Indicative of this situation was the response of James Chin, former director of the infectious diseases program for the California Department of Health Services, and his colleague Donald Francis to the assertion that their recommendation that HIV-infected women not become pregnant — included as part of a broad strategy of prevention — was "directive" (Chin and Francis 1987). For them the charge was unwarranted, since they never questioned the ultimate right of infected women to choose whether or not to become pregnant. That, they believed, was at the heart of the "nondirective" posture which they, too, endorsed (Francis and Chin 1987). Given the extent to which public health officials, and especially those with primary responsibility for the protection of maternal and child health, had either explicitly or implicitly absorbed the ideology of nondirective counseling, the reaction to the prospects of the birth of HIV-infected infants was all the more striking.

AIDS and Counseling for Prevention

When the Centers for Disease Control (CDC) first addressed the problem of vertical transmission of HIV infection in December 1985, it spoke directly about the importance of identifying women at risk. The broad spectrum of clinical settings through which such women passed was to offer voluntary testing and counseling. The purpose was clear: the prevention of the birth of infected babies. "Infected women should be advised to consider delaying pregnancy until more is known about perinatal transmission of the virus" (Centers for Disease Control 1985, 725). The case for testing pregnant women, put forth with equal vigor by the CDC, was less clear, since for political reasons the option of abortion could not even be mentioned (Grimes 1987). Such silence was especially ironic since only counseling informed pregnant women about the option of abortion and making the termination of pregnancy a possibility for those who chose such a course could serve the preventive goals of the CDC. Made at a time when relatively little was known about the actual risks of transmission for infected women to their fetuses, the recommendation that women be urged to consider forgoing pregnancy represented a determination to apply standard public health norms to the reproductive realm. In the face of uncertainty, prevention required the adoption of a posture of caution. What made this stance unusual was the reticence that convention had dictated in matters affecting the substance of reproductive choice.

To some extent this break with accepted norms may be explained by the professional backgrounds of the CDC officials most responsible for formulating AIDS policy. It was venereal disease control, rather than the delicate question of how to face the matter of relative risk in the face of reproductive decisions, that informed their thinking. Indeed, they never seriously considered the relevance of the large and complex literature on nondirective genetic counseling to the problem of pediatric AIDS (James Allen, personal communication). But they did not long remain unaware of that alternative perspective. At least three of the consultants brought together by the CDC to consider its draft recommendations warned of the potential abuses that might follow from an explicit effort to discourage pregnancy.

Janet Mitchell, a black obstetrician and perinatologist, noted the history of coercive reproductive practices faced by minority women in public hospitals (Lori Andrews, personal communication). Advice, she feared, would ineluctably take on restrictive dimensions. Both Lori Andrews, a specialist on the legal aspects of reproduction on the staff of the American Bar Foundation, and Leroy Walters, a medical ethicist, urged the adoption of the genetic counseling model in the framing of public policy on perinatal HIV infection. To those pleas the response was one of incredulity. "Don't you want to stop the spread of AIDS to infants?" they were asked by CDC officials.

The language adopted by the CDC was somewhat tentative in form. Women were advised to *consider* the *delaying* of pregnancy. (Virtually all discussion of vertical HIV transmission focuses on women; rarely are infected men a subject of discussion.) Suggesting a "delay" of pregnancy conveyed a less drastic impression of what was, in fact, being called for. Since the available scientific evidence made clear that HIV infection was lifelong, it was not a postponement but a forgoing of pregnancy that was required by the preventive orientation. Further-more, by urging women to "consider" a fundamental curtailment of their reproductive lives it appeared that the CDC was not itself coun-seling women to make such a choice. Nevertheless, there can be no doubt about how the CDC believed women ought to act in the face of HIV infection. In virtually every statement by officials since the De-cember 1985 recommendations were published in *Morbidity and Mor-tality Weekly Report*, the preventive goal has been put forth bluntly. Speaking about the logic of testing and counseling, James Curran, di-rector of AIDS activities at the CDC, stated: "There is no reason that the number of [pediatric AIDS cases] shouldn't decline. . . . Someone who understands the disease and is logical will not want to be pregnant and will consider the test results when making family planning deci-sions" (*CDC AIDS Weekly* 1988). If anything, Curran's CDC colleague Martha Rogers was more direct in addressing the challenge of vertical HIV transmission. Women and their sexual partners would have to "suppress often strong desires to bear children" (Rogers 1987, 109).

State, and some local, health departments have in a variety of ways adopted the substance of the CDC's recommendations on vertical HIV transmission as their own. (These data are based on a survey of state health departments; information on policy was conveyed in the form of personal communications and copies of state policy statements.) Across the nation, in locales with virtually no cases of pediatric AIDS as well as in those with relatively high levels of maternal transmission, in juris-dictions that have stressed the importance of protecting the privacy and social interests of the infected and those that have been less concerned with such matters, the goal of preventing the birth of infected babies has been explicitly embraced by public health officials. Like the CDC, state health departments have typically remained circumspect about the role of testing in pregnant women. In a few instances the possibility of abortion has been mentioned. In no case were women urged to ter-minate their pregnancies or even urged to consider such procedures.

Although virtually all states have spoken about postponing preg-nancy, only a few have adopted the CDC's circumspect formulation that urged women to "consider" such a course. New Jersey, with its heavy burden of pediatric AIDS cases, has done so. Far more common has been the more straightforward recommendation that "women post-pone or avoid pregnancy for the time being." Michigan, for example, has "strongly encouraged [infected women] to delay pregnancy." The

San Francisco Health Department, so exquisitely sensitive to the ethical problems posed by counseling and to the rights of infected men, was equally blunt. "Whenever possible, women infected with HIV should be confidentially identified and educated about the risks of perinatal transmission. Infected women should be advised to postpone pregnancy. . . . [Pregnant women] should be counseled to postpone subsequent pregnancies" (Rutherford et al. 1987, 105). In many cases, health departments have ignored the subtle equivocation in the CDC's phrasing and have declared: "We follow the recommendations of the CDC and urge women not to become pregnant."

In at least two instances states have employed both the tentative formulation used by the CDC as well as more overtly directive language, suggesting thereby institutional tensions and ambivalence. Addressing the physicians of New York State in July 1985, the commissioner of health recommended that infected women postpone pregnancy. In January 1988 the state's "Guide to Physicians on Counseling and Testing Women of Childbearing Age" adopted the less-directive CDC formulation. In the same month, however, a health department brochure meant for distribution in family planning clinics stated: "Having a baby? Have a test for the AIDS virus first. . . . If you have the AIDS virus: Postpone pregnancy to protect your baby and you. . . ."

In Massachusetts even greater confusion reigned in 1988. The commissioner of health stated: "While the AIDS office urges all women to be aware and concerned about possible transmission and its consequences, there is *no* policy in place to direct women to make any one choice over the other" (Deborah Prothrow-Stith, personal communication). This nondirective posture, so consistent with the prevailing model of genetic counseling, was reflected in a health department pamphlet, "Women, Babies and AIDS," which never even suggested postponement of pregnancy as an option. Nevertheless, another state-produced brochure, "Family Planning Facts about AIDS," asserted: "Women with positive test results should not get pregnant until more is known about HIV infection and pregnancy."

Support for the systematic effort to discourage pregnancy in HIV-infected women came also from professionals involved in maternal and child health as well as from their professional associations. At the April 1987 Surgeon General's Workshop on Children with HIV Infection and Their Families, the task force charged with the responsibility for developing recommendations on reducing the risks of maternal/fetal transmission explicitly urged that infected women be "advised to defer pregnancy," although it noted the "difficulties" that would be faced by many women who might consider such a course. Two months later the Committee on Obstetrics, Maternal and Fetal Medicine and Gynecologic Practice of the American College of Obstetrics and Gynecology (1987) published a report stating that infected women "should be strongly encouraged not to become pregnant and should be provided with appropriate family planning assistance." The college's *Technical Bulletin*, which serves as a professional standard of practice, adopted a similar stance in 1988, stressing that infected women should be discouraged from becoming pregnant. Not hobbled by the political constraints impinging upon recommendations of many public health officials, the *Technical Bulletin* could state that HIV-infected pregnant women should be informed about their reproductive options, including elective abortions.

How much such positions reflect the beliefs of practitioners, obstetricians, and nonmedical counselors, and how effective such statements have been in helping to shape their beliefs and practices, is not yet known. Some reports suggest that, at least insofar as physicians are concerned, a directive approach to both the question of the postponement and termination of pregnancy has begun to emerge. Dismay about the willingness of infected women to carry their pregnancies to term has been evident to some who continue to urge a traditional nondirective counseling posture. "People are not going to admit [publicly] they're doing directive counseling. But we all know it's being done" (Abraham 1988). In a survey of two pediatric residency programs in New York City, 65 percent of the respondents "agreed" or "strongly agreed" with the proposition that "women should not have babies who will be at risk for [AIDS]." That was true for only 25 percent when the risk was for Tay-Sachs disease, and 15 percent when the risk was for cystic fibrosis — both leading to painful and tragically shortened juvenile lives — and 9 percent when the risk was for Down's syndrome. It is not surprising, therefore, that 43 percent of the respondents would mandate the testing of pregnant women, and that the remaining 57 percent believed that women should be directively counseled to undergo testing. None of the respondents believed that nondirective counseling for antibody testing was appropriate (Betty Levin, personal communication).

Physicians had always been more directive in their approach to reproductive matters than had nonmedical counselors in a way that reflected the conventional practice of medicine. But these data suggest much more. The study's respondents had clearly indicated a greater willingness to adopt a directive posture with regard to AIDS than with other grave genetic disorders. It is possible that both the class and racial/ethnic background of those at risk for transmitting HIV infection played a critical role. That so many infected women were also intravenous drug users may also have been a significant factor. But whatever motivated the responses of those surveyed, it is clear that the disquiet provoked by pediatric AIDS had elicited a willingness to embrace, in a remarkable way, clinical practices that deviated from the conventions of nondirective counseling.

Among those working in the field of bioethics, there has been a notable reluctance to apply formulaic responses to the issue of maternal HIV transmission. Despite the nondirective posture conventionally adopted in matters involving severe genetic disorders including Tay-Sachs (Elias and Annas 1987), a number of philosophers (e.g., John Arras, personal communication) and lawyers have asserted that they were troubled by efforts to denounce as unethical attempts to discourage pregnancy among infected women. The "harm principle," which provides a moral limit on the exercise of freedom when others may be injured, has emerged as a countervailing force to conceptions of autonomy that had heretofore treated directive counseling as a threat to free choice.

Nothing more tellingly reveals the extent to which the threat of perinatal HIV infection had generated an urgent preventive posture than the response of the March of Dimes. Established in 1938 to combat polio, the organization had in 1958 redefined its mission to include the prevention of birth defects. Out of its own organizational and professional history, but especially as a consequence of its desire to distinguish sharply between a commitment to the preventions of birth defects and an endorsement of abortion, a strong ideological commitment to preserving the reproductive freedom of those served by recipients of its grants emerged. Indeed, it adopted a policy that explicitly forbade its grantees from directively counseling those at risk for bearing children with defects (March of Dimes Birth Defects Foundation 1973). In its public campaign to prevent the birth of babies with HIV infection—conducted in brochures as well as television spots—the March of Dimes urged women at risk to be tested before pregnancy so that they might make "informed decisions." But despite the emphasis on permitting women to make their own choices, there could be little mistake about how the March of Dimes believed those choices should be made. "A baby born with AIDS is born dying," states the off-camera voice as the strings supporting a baby-like marionette are cut by a pair of scissors (March of Dimes Birth Defects Foundation 1988).

Despite the broad-based support for efforts to identify HIV-infected women so that they might be counseled and discouraged from becoming pregnant, the conventional nondirective posture has been given voice by feminist critics of the emerging consensus. For them the alacrity with which public health officials and clinicians had embraced the goal of dissuading HIV-infected women from becoming pregnant was in large measure a reflection of the willingness to override the preferences of poor black and Hispanic women who had always been vulnerable to the pressure of white professional men. A woman's right to choose had to be preserved despite the risks associated with AIDS. Those who were not pregnant had a right to counseling that would permit them to make choices unencumbered by directive interventions. Those who were pregnant had a right to bear a child or to abort. Directive counseling would inevitably entail elements of subtle coercion and might ineluctably lead to more blatant forms of pressure. Only non-directive counseling—whatever its limits—would preclude the subversion of reproductive rights. This perspective was captured by the Supreme Court at a moment when the liberal majority that had crafted the ruling in *Roe v. Wade* still held sway. "Counseling about pregnancy outcome must not be conducted in such a way that its goal is less to inform than to influence which option the woman should choose."[1] The fears provoked by the tone and substance of public policy on vertical transmission of HIV infection extended beyond the issue of AIDS, however. Animating the deeply felt anxiety was the concern that the carefully wrought but always vulnerable ideology of reproductive freedom could be subject to a severe insult by the effort to control the spread of HIV infection. Those fears were intensified by the political vigor of the antiabortion movement, the receptivity of elected officials to its demands, and the very clear indications, even prior to *Webster* that the Supreme Court might be willing to reconsider or fundamentally circumscribe its 1973 abortion ruling.

If feminists and their political allies were troubled by the possibility

---

[1] *Akron Center for Reproductive Health v. City of Akron*, 462 U.S. 416 (1983).

of the erosion of women's rights, those whose perspective was shaped
by concerns for the rights of women of color responded to the call for
reproductive restraint with the memories of compulsory sterilization
abuse all too fresh (Proctor 1988). The even more recent debacle associated with mandatory sickle-cell screening also framed their reaction.
Among the most forceful critics of the public health posture on HIV
infection and pregnancy was Janet Mitchell. Centering her challenge on
the failure of those counseling deferral of pregnancy to appreciate the
cultural and social contexts of reproductive choice and on their failure
to understand the very different ways in which professional, often
white, counselors and poor, often black and Hispanic, women understood the meaning of relative risk, she has underscored the importance
of procreation to the women in whose defense she has written. For intravenous drug-using women the counsel of restraint was portrayed as
especially "devastating," threatening to deprive them of what hope
they had for a better life. "We forget that those women have a strong
innate need to procreate. . . . We must be cautious in how we approach our need to do good, to do no harm." For Mitchell (1988, 51)
the central issue forced by the public health assertion that HIV-infected
women should avoid pregnancy "is the right of every woman to reproductive self-determination, regardless of her station in life." More stri-
dently, the claim that the risk of bearing an HIV-infected baby should
lead all infected women to forgo pregnancy has been termed by some
a strategy for racial depopulation, as genocidal (Helen Gasch, personal
communication).

AIDS and the Future of
Reproductive Choice

Despite the well-established convention of nondirective counseling in
reproductive matters, as a matter of both professional ideology and
practice, there is no question but that counselors have — at times more
frequently than most would find comfortable to acknowledge — sought
to press women at risk to follow a particular course. In recent years
some clinicians and academic commentators have publicly argued the
case for directive counseling for those at high risk for genetic disorders
such as Huntington's chorea. But those who have broken ranks with
the conventions of reproductive counseling have done so virtually al-

ways as individuals challenging those conventions. What makes the prevailing situation regarding perinatally acquired HIV infection so striking is that professional associations of medical practitioners and public health agencies at federal and state levels have adopted a directive posture. There has been, therefore, a dramatic reversal of the institutional context of the public discussion. What can account for this rupture with convention?

It is, of course, possible that those charting public policy on pediatric AIDS have thought about it differently because of the language of crisis that has surrounded virtually every dimension of the epidemic. Furthermore, concern about the potential social costs that would be incurred by the care of HIV-infected babies may have contributed to the sense of urgency. From a public health perspective it was not a very long step from the directive advice given to those who were infected about the necessity of changed sexual and needle-sharing behavior to directive advice about becoming pregnant, if not about the course to follow if already pregnant.

Contributing to the climate within which the determination to discourage pregnancy among HIV-infected women was made, and the response with which it was greeted by many of those who had so forcefully defended the ethos of unencumbered individual reproductive choice by women, was the broad-based challenge to the ideological hegemony of individualism in American society. It was no longer cultural conservatives alone who raised questions about the intellectual, social, moral, and political consequences of a liberalism so individualistic in its commitments. Within bioethics the almost singular devotion to "rights" and autonomy has come under repeated attack that extends arguments first made by foundational figures such as Daniel Callahan (1981), William May (1975), and Leon Kass (1985). Feminist thinkers, too, have been compelled to confront the limits of individualism as they face the question of maternal surrogacy and amniocentesis for gender selection. Finally, advances in genetic diagnosis have revitalized eugenic thinking, permitting a challenge to the orthodoxies of genetic counseling. Nothing more tellingly reveals the current receptivity to critiques of individualism than the warm response accorded to *Habits of the Heart* by Robert Bellah et al. (1985), a volume that so forcefully and imaginatively argued the case for a renewal of a communitarian perspective.

The willingness of public health officials to urge infected women not to become pregnant must also be understood in the light of an emerg-

ing trend of seeking to compel pregnant women to undergo medical
treatments in order to protect the lives of their fetuses (Nelson and
Milliken 1988). One study reported on 21 cases in which court orders
were sought to override maternal refusals of such therapy. Permission
was granted in all but three cases. When the directors of maternal/fetal
medicine fellowship programs were questioned, just less than one-half
believed that women who defied medical advice, ᵗhus endangering
their fetuses, should be detained for medical supervision. Similar
proportions believed that court orders should be sought for intrauterine
transfusions. Less than one-quarter of the respondents consistently upheld the right of competent women to refuse medical advice. To the
authors of the report, the implications of the trend for the full range of
the rights of pregnant women were all too clear (Kolder, Gallagher,
and Parsons 1987). For George Annas (1987, 1213) the instances of coercive treatment suggested an ominous turn: "The beginning of an alliance between physicians and the state to force pregnant women to
follow medical advice for the sake of their fetuses."

The possibility of such an alliance haunts the discussion of the potential impact of efforts to prevent the birth of infants with AIDS.
Will the adoption of a directive posture on perinatal HIV transmission
contribute to current attempts to circumscribe the reproductive rights
of women? Will they foster a climate within which eugenic perspectives
will be given added legitimacy? Although historically linked, the social
forces seeking to restrict reproductive freedom and those advancing eugenic goals now have been uncoupled. Indeed, the social forces that
may succeed in achieving the former may attain their goals at the expense of the latter.

The contemporary movement against the unrestricted reproductive
freedom of women has, especially through the influence of the Roman
Catholic Church, a pronatalist dimension. Opposed to abortion, it contains also an important constituency that is hostile to the compulsory
sterilization of women. It is thus unlikely that the threat of maternal
HIV transmission will result in a politically effective campaign for compulsory sterilization, or coerced abortion. As strategies of prevention,
such efforts would not only confront the opposition of those who have
struggled to protect the reproductive rights of women but of their bitter opponents in the antiabortion movement as well. Against such an
alliance no "public health" drive to prohibit surgically the birth of babies with HIV infection is likely to achieve broad-based political sup-

port. It is, however, possible that some local efforts will be made to criminalize the birth of HIV-infected babies. Such moves might derive their intellectual justification from the proposals to punish women who bear children with severe genetic disorders (Shaw 1984), and might derive political support from aggressive prosecutors who have so recently sought to indict drug-addicted women who have given birth to addicted babies.

The prospects are greater for a contribution to the advancement of the eugenic perspective. Historically, the eugenics movement had sought to restrict procreation on the part of those who might bear "defective" children who would, in turn, contribute to racial degeneration by having children who would further pollute the genetic pool. But concern about the propagation of undesirable genetic material has not been the only concern. At times eugenicists have sought to prevent the birth of those with disorders, however unlikely the prospect that they in turn would bear children. The prospect of the birth of children who would pose a social burden, of those who, because of their handicaps, would never be able to attain economic independence was sufficient to provoke an interest in restrictive policies. The eugenic world view has thus been extended to include "any effort to interfere with individuals' procreative choices to attain a societal goal" (Perutz 1989, 35). It is within such a broadly conceptualized eugenic outlook that efforts to convince HIV-infected women to forgo pregnancy must be understood.

There are, of course, critical differences among procreative policies that would systematically seek to enforce a program of communal enhancement, those that would seek to discourage women or couples from choosing to bear children when the risks of severe disability are high, and those that would enhance the likelihood that women will bear healthy children with the fewest impediments to fulfilling lives. Rarely do those with eugenic commitments today propose the enactment of laws that would deprive at-risk individuals of the freedom to procreate. Rather, as in the case of HIV infection, they tend to stress the role of persuasion—sometimes quite aggressive—and public education even for the best in utero care of the fetus. Nevertheless, even a noncoercive eugenics could have profound and often troubling consequences. A eugenic ethos might not only affect the ways in which individuals would choose to exercise their reproductive options, but the social tolerance for those born less than perfect, including the way in which those with congenital disorders might be treated by the health care system, the extent to which the cost of providing such care would be viewed as too socially burdensome, the prospect of treating impaired newborns, and perhaps including them as prime candidates for "rationing." Proponents of policies with eugenic implications cannot avoid a serious consideration of such issues, however benign their intentions.

Whether the eugenic dimensions of current policies designed to limit the birth of infants with AIDS will contribute to a climate of social intolerance for those with HIV infection, and whether such policies will contribute to a more general climate of intolerance for those with disabilities and genetic disorders, will in large measure depend on the balance of political, social, and intellectual forces far broader than those directly linked to the epidemic. AIDS is but a small part of the medical, political, and ideological context within which contemporary controversies over eugenics are being waged. Indeed, the very uniqueness of the HIV epidemic may serve to circumscribe the impact of policies adopted to prevent its spread.

But whatever the ultimate impact of effort to prevent the maternal transmission of HIV infection, the broadly shared preventive impulse provoked by pediatric AIDS has provided yet another instance of the inadequacy of the prevailing ideological underpinnings of the commitment to reproductive freedom. The limits of liberal individualism, which has sought to shield procreative decisions from restrictive social and moral judgments, have become increasingly apparent even to those who have drawn upon its force to press for social and political reform. The question that now presents itself is whether it will be possible, under contemporary political conditions, to frame an ideological perspective that will transcend those limits without calling forth the very conditions against which liberalism represented such a liberating challenge, that will be capable of informing the public culture within which women will make their decisions about reproduction.

References

Abraham, L. 1988. Pregnant Women Face AIDS Dilemma. *American Medical News* (July 22):3, 34–35.

American College of Obstetrics and Gynecology. 1988. *AIDS Technical Bulletin*. Washington.

Annas, G. 1987. Protecting the Liberty of Pregnant Patients. *New England Journal of Medicine* 316(19):1213–14.

Asch, A. 1989. Reproductive Technology and Disability. In *Reproductive Laws for the 1990s*, ed. S. Cohen and N. Taub, 69–124. Clifton, N.J.: Humana Press.

Bayer, R. 1989. *Private Acts, Social Consequences: AIDS and the Politics of Public Health*. New York: Free Press.

Bellah, R. N., R. Madsen, W.M. Sullivan, A. Swidler, and S.M. Tipton. 1985. *Habits of the Heart*. New York: Harper and Row.

Bird, S. 1985. Presymptomatic Testing for Huntington's Disease. *Journal of the American Medical Association* 253(22):3286–91.

Callahan, D. 1981. Minimalist Ethics. *Hastings Center Report* 11(5):19–25.

Callahan, S. 1979. An Ethical Analysis of Responsible Parenthood. In *Genetic Counseling: Facts, Values and Norms*, ed. A. Capron, M. Lappe, R. Murray, T. Powledge, S. Twiss, and D. Bergman, 217–238. New York: Alan Liss.

CDC AIDS Weekly. October 3, 1988. Curran Supports Testing, Counseling for Pregnant Women.

Centers for Disease Control. 1985. Recommendations for Assisting in the Prevention of Perinatal Transmission of Human T-Lymphotropic Virus Type III/Lymphodenopathy-Associated Virus and Acquired Immunodeficiency Syndrome. *Morbidity and Mortality Weekly Report* 34:721–32.

———. 1989. *HIV/AIDS Surveillance* (March). Atlanta.

Chin, J., and D. Francis. 1987. The Prevention of Acquired Immunodeficiency Syndrome in the United States: An Objective Strategy for Medicine, Public Health, Business and the Community. *Journal of the American Medical Association* 257(10):1357–66.

Committee on Obstetrics, Maternal and Fetal Medicine and Gynecologic Practice of the American College of Obstetrics and Gynecology. 1987. *Prevention of Human Immunodeficiency Virus Infection and Acquired Immune Deficiency Syndrome*. Washington.

Edelman, R., and H. Haverkos. 1989. The Suitability of HIV Positive Individuals for Marriage and Pregnancy. *Journal of the American Medical Association* 261(7):993.

Elias, S., and G. Annas. 1987. *Reproductive Genetics and the Law*. Chicago: Year Book Medical Publishers.

Fletcher, J.F. 1980. Knowledge, Risk and the Right to Reproduce. In *Genetics and the Law II*, ed. A. Milunsky and G.J. Annas, 187–209. New York: Plenum Press.

Francis, D., and J. Chin. 1987. Counseling the HIV-positive Woman Regarding Pregnancy. *Journal of the American Medical Association* 257(24):3361.

Fraser, F. 1974. Genetic Counseling. *Journal of Human Genetics* 26:636–59.

Grimes, D. 1987. The CDC and Abortion of HIV-Positive Women. *Journal of the American Medical Association* 258(9):1176.

Haverkos, H. and Edelman, R. 1988. The Epidemiology of Acquired Immunodeficiency Syndrome Among Heterosexuals. *Journal of the American Medical Association* 260(13):1922–1929.

Hoskins, B., and H. Holmes. 1984. Technology and Prenatal Femicide. In *Test Tube Women*, ed. R. Klein and S. Minden, 237–55. London: Pandora Press.

Hubbard, R. 1988. A Feminist Views Prenatal Diagnosis. *Newsletter of the National Society of Genetic Counselors.* 10(2):1.

Institute of Society, Ethics, and the Life Sciences. 1972. Ethical and Social Issues in Screening for Genetic Disease. *New England Journal of Medicine* 286(25):1129–32.

Karst, K. 1980. The Freedom of Intimate Association. *Yale Law Journal* 89(1):624–92.

Kass, L. 1985. *Toward a More Natural Science: Biology and Human Affairs.* New York: Free Press.

Katz Rothman, B. 1986. *The Tentative Pregnancy.* New York: Viking Press.

Kevles, D. 1985. *In the Name of Eugenics.* New York: Knopf.

Kolder, V., J. Gallagher, and M. Parsons. 1987. Court Ordered Obstetrical Interventions. *New England Journal of Medicine* 316(19):1192–96.

Landesman, S., A. Willoughby, and H. Minkoff. 1989. HIV Disease in Reproductive Age Women: A Problem of the Present. *Journal of the American Medical Association* 261(9):1326–27.

Ludmerer, K. 1972. *Genetics and American Society.* Baltimore: Johns Hopkins University Press.

March of Dimes Birth Defects Foundation. 1973. *Policies and Procedures Governing Medical Service Grants.* White Plains, N.Y.

————. 1988. *Born Dying.* White Plains, N.Y.

May, W. 1975. Code, Covenant, Contract or Philanthropy. *Hastings Center Report* 5(6):29–38.

Mitchell, J.L. 1988. Women, AIDS and Public Policy. *AIDS and Public Policy Journal* 3(2):50–52.

National Academy of Sciences. 1975. *Genetic Screening: Programs, Principles and Research.* Washington: Academy Press.

Nelkin, D., and L. Tancredi. 1989. *Dangerous Diagnostics: The Social Power of Biological Information.* New York: Basic Books.

Nelson, L., and J. Milliken. 1988. Compelled Medical Treatment of Pregnant Women. *Journal of the American Medical Association* 259(7):1060–66.

Novick, L., D. Berns, R. Stricof, R. Stevens, K. Pass, and J. Wethers. 1989. HIV Seroprevalence in Newborns in New York State. *Journal of the American Medical Association* 261(12):1745–50.

Perry, T. 1981. Some Ethical Problems in Huntington's Chorea. *Canadian Medical Journal* 125:1098–1100.

Perutz, M. 1989. Should Genes Be Screened? *New York Review of Books* (May 18):34–36. Citing *Proceed with Caution: Predicting Genetic Risks in the Recombinant DNA Era* by N. Holtzman. Baltimore: Johns Hopkins University Press.

Petchesky, R. 1984. *Abortion and a Woman's Right to Choose.* New York: Longman.

President's Commission on Ethical Problems in Medicine and Biomedical and Behavioral Research. 1982. *Screening and Counseling for Genetic Conditions.* Washington.

Proctor, R. 1988. *Racial Hygiene: Medicine under the Nazis.* Cambridge: Harvard University Press.

Rapp, R. 1988. Chromosomes and Communication: The Discourse of Genetic Counseling. *Medical Anthropology Quarterly* 2(2):143-57.

Reed, S. 1974. A Short History of Genetic Counseling. *Social Biology* 21(4): 331-39.

Report of the Surgeon General's Workshop on Children with HIV Infection and their Families. 1987. Washington.

Rogers, M. 1987. Controlling Perinatally Acquired HIV Infection. *Western Journal of Medicine* 147:109-10.

Rose, H. 1987. The Politics of Reproductive Science. In *Reproductive Technologies*, ed. M. Stanworth, 155-73. Minneapolis: University of Minnesota Press.

Rutherford, G.E., M. Grossman, J.R. Green, D.W. Wara, N.S. Shaw, D.F. Echenberg, C.B. Wofsy, D.H. Weinstein, F. Stroud, E.S. Sarsfield, and D. Werdegar. 1987. Guidelines for the Control of Perinatally Transmitted Human Immunodeficiency Virus Infection and Care of Infected Mothers. *Western Journal of Medicine* 147:104-8.

Ruzek, S. 1978. *The Women's Health Movement: Feminist Alternatives to Medical Control.* New York: Praeger.

Selwyn, P., E.E. Schoenbaum, K.D. Davenny, V.J. Robertson, A.R. Feingold, J.S. Schulman, M.M. Mayers, R.S. Klein, G.H. Friedland, and M.F. Rogers. 1989. Prospective Study of Human Immunodeficiency Virus Infection and Pregnancy Outcomes in Intravenous Drug Users. *Journal of the American Medical Association* 261(9):1289-94.

Shaw, M.W. 1984. Conditional Prospective Rights of the Fetus. *Journal of Legal Medicine* 5(1):63-116.

Sorenson, J.R., J. Swazey, and N.A. Scotch. 1981. *Reproductive Pasts, Reproductive Futures.* New York: Alan Liss.

Stanworth, M. 1987. Reproductive Technologies and the Deconstruction of Motherhood. In *Reproductive Technologies*, ed. M. Stanworth. Minneapolis: University of Minnesota Press.

Sunderland, A., G. Moroso, M. Berthaud, S. Holman, F. Cancellieri, H. Mendez, S. Landesman, and H. Minkoff. 1988. Influence of HIV Infection on Pregnancy Decisions, *Fourth International Conference on AIDS, Stockholm, Sweden, Abstract 6607.*

Wertz, D., and J. Fletcher. 1988. Attitudes of Genetic Counselors: A Multinational Survey. *American Journal of Human Genetics* 42:592-600.

Wikler, N. 1986. Society's Response to the New Reproductive Technologies: The Feminist Perspective. *Southern California Law Review* 59(5):1043-57.

World Health Organization. 1968. *Screening for Inborn Errors of Metabolism.* Technical Reprint Series no. 401. Geneva.

Acknowledgments: Work on this chapter was supported by a grant from the Conanima Foundation, the Josiah Macy, Jr. Foundation, and the American Foundation for AIDS Research.

The Poisoned Gift
AIDS and Blood

THOMAS H. MURRAY

D R. LOUISE KEATING BECAME "TRASH CZAR" FOR
a few days. Dr. Keating, director of Red Cross Blood Services
in Cleveland, found her center almost engulfed by mounds of
debris—dressings, needles, plastic tubes—most of it the usual detritus
of any organization, but some of it splashed with the blood of donors.
Her center was not generating any more trash than usual. But suddenly
no one was willing to cart it away. AIDS could be transmitted through
blood, we had now learned. Last year's innocuous garbage had become
this year's plague vector. Or so it seemed to Cleveland's carters. And
the refuse piles grew.

Dr. Keating did solve her problem. Now, all waste that has any
blood on it is sterilized in an autoclave until nothing, not even a virus,
survives. But AIDS has created many other problems in the nation's
blood supply: for those, like Dr. Keating and her colleagues, who must
find donors and ensure that the blood obtained is safe; for those who
give blood; and for those who receive it.

We live in a community that has chosen to provide for its members'
needs for whole blood by a system of gifts. Donors receive no monetary
compensation for their blood; recipients are charged for the costs of obtaining, testing, storing, and transporting the blood, but not a "sup-
plier's" fee. In a culture that deems markets the proper means to
produce and distribute goods and that celebrates self-interest as the

216

wellspring of human action, gifts of blood may seem anomalous and mysterious. With the knowledge that the human immunodeficiency virus (HIV) can be transmitted through blood came the realization that such a gift might be poisoned. This chapter is an attempt to understand the moral significance of that realization and its implications for the donation of blood and for the concepts of community that gifts of blood represent.

While we do not know how many people have been infected with HIV through blood or blood products, we do have reliable estimates of the numbers diagnosed with AIDS. According to the Centers for Disease Control (CDC), as of January 1990, a total of 4,346 people with AIDS probably contracted it by receiving blood or blood products (such as the clotting factors needed by people with hemophilia or other clotting disorders). Of these, 2,922 adults and 217 children had been infected with AIDS through whole blood or blood components, while 1,099 adults and 108 children received it through clotting factors derived from blood. This amounts to 4 percent of the total cases of AIDS in the United States (Centers for Disease Control 1990).

With these data in mind, I want to trace some of the impact that AIDS has had on the donation of blood and other gifts of the body. The effects I refer to — some of which are subtle, others perhaps more pervasive and significant — can only be described in terms of the meaning and importance of these anonymous and often life-saving gifts to strangers. To understand the nature of such a system of gifts we must recover a pair of seemingly anachronistic ideas, and the languages that permit their description and justification: the ideas of gift and of community.

Gifts and Community

The contemporary "gift shop" makes the practice of gift exchange easy and routine. A selection of items, usually pleasant or pretty, rarely useful, is displayed so that the buyer can find an appropriate trinket quickly. Efficient and pleasant, the gift shop tries to make the potentially onerous duty of selecting the right gift as painless as possible.

The gift shop facilitates two superficially contradictory facets of our attitude toward gifts: our desire to make the giving of them efficient and easy (so what if items cost more in gift boutiques; our time is worth something!) and the lingering importance of gifts as a mode of social relations (if gift exchange were insignificant, then we would not feel the need to sustain the rhythm of receiving and giving). But there is no actual contradiction here, merely a failure to understand fully the significance of gift exchange in contemporary life. Because we underestimate the importance of gifts, perhaps we flee too readily to the modern institution that offers to "solve the problem" of gift exchange.

Our currently thin understanding of gifts has deep historical roots. By 1767, the renowned legal commentator William Blackstone (1715–1769) had written that "gifts are always gratuitous" and require "no consideration or equivalent." Gifts were thus distinguished from other modes of social exchange in which something was indeed expected from the receiving party. This meaning of gift as derived from law is reflected in the definition offered by the *Oxford English Dictionary*: "the transference of property in a thing by one person to another, voluntarily and without any valuable consideration." Gifts, in this perspective, do not spring from any obligations, nor do they impose any. They are the blithe and free spirits of property transfer.

Not everyone has portrayed gifts in such a benign and trifling manner. To Ralph Waldo Emerson ([1844] 1979), gifts were pernicious. In his essay "Gifts" he wrote: "It is not the office of a man to receive gifts. How dare you give them? We wish to be self-sustained. We do not quite forgive a giver."

Is it possible to reconcile these two apparently antithetic meanings of gift? I believe it is, through an understanding of the role gifts have played in other cultures and at other times.

The locus classicus for anthropologic discussions of gifts is Marcel Mauss's ([1925] 1967) *Essai sur le don, forme archaïque de l'échange*. Mauss analyzed patterns of exchange among peoples in Melanesia, Polynesia, and the Pacific Northwest. Groups within these regions exchanged many objects — sacred objects such as elaborately decorated copper ornaments, shell necklaces, and bracelets, as well as feasts, festivals, entertainments, and other social events. In the rhythm of giving and receiving, Mauss found a powerful glue that held disparate tribes, clans, and phratries together in peace despite the ever-present forces pressing for conflict: fear of that which was different, suspicion, resentment.

The first modern myth dispelled by Mauss was that gifts were, as Blackstone's description implied, things freely given and imposing no obligations on the recipient. In reality, gifts are permeated with obligation. While the "opening gift" may be given in comparative freedom, once a gift is given in return the givers/receivers become enmeshed in a never-resting cycle of offering and accepting. In every culture examined, Mauss found that gifts are typically given out of a perceived obligation or necessity, and that they, in return, impose strenuous obligations on recipients.

Another myth is that gifts are always given altruistically and disinterestedly. To the contrary, among the peoples Mauss studied, gifts serve crucial social needs, especially the need to establish bonds among people who might otherwise be in conflict. For the Trobrianders, gifts circulate continuously and in two directions: *mwali*, ceremonial armshells, and *soulava*, necklaces of red spondylus shell. This never-ceasing cycle of gifts is called *kula*, which translates as "ring." Mauss ([1925] 1967, 20) writes that "it seems as if all these tribes, the sea journeys, the precious objects, the food and feasts, the economic, ritual and sexual services, the men and the women, were caught in a ring around which they kept up a regular movement in time and space." *Kula* is a ring that unites the Dobu, Kiriwana, Sinaketa, and other tribes—a circle within which peace reigns and commerce is possible.

Gifts serve purposes other than the efficient transfer of useful goods. The early anthropologist Alfred Radcliffe-Brown recognized this in his study of the people of North Andaman:

> The exchange of presents did not serve the same purpose as trade or barter in more developed communities. The purpose that it did serve was a moral one. The object of the exchange was to produce a friendly feeling between the two persons concerned, and unless it did this it failed of its purpose (Mauss [1925] 1967, 18).

Mauss ([1925] 1967, 31) describes how the exchange of gifts is much more than the trade of objects because "the objects are never completely separated from the men who exchange them; the communion and alliance they establish are well-nigh indissoluble" and contribute to the way such groups "are constantly embroiled with and feel themselves in debt to each other."

Gifts are objects or events given not for their own sake, but for the sake of the relations between the tribes, clans, other groups—or individuals. Mauss ([1925] 1967, 11) expresses it with characteristic bluntness:

"To refuse to give, or to fail to invite, is—like refusing to accept—the equivalent of a declaration of war; it is a refusal of friendship and intercourse." Understanding this concept affords some insight into the confusion—to our minds—between the gift-objects and the people who gave them common among the people Mauss studied. Describing the powerful and elaborate rights and duties that characterize gifts, Mauss ([1925] 1967, 11) claims that "the pattern . . . is not difficult to understand if we realize that it is first and foremost a pattern of spiritual bonds between things which are to some extent parts of persons." In blood and other modern gifts of the body, the gifts are literally, not merely symbolically, parts of persons.

Gifts have, as Lewis Hyde (1983) puts it, an "erotic" force, erotic in the sense of attraction, union, that which binds together. This force is most evident in our intimate relations with family and friends. We use gifts to sustain relationships and to initiate them. A norm of reciprocity governs gifts, requiring that gifts be exchanged, and that they be of comparable or greater value where the means of the parties are similar. The roughly equal value of goods exchanged may make it appear as if something much like a contract was at work, but this is to misunderstand the fundamental contrast between gift and contract. Contracts facilitate the trading of something—objects, services, promises; the relationship created by the contract is merely a means to that end. Gifts facilitate the creation and sustaining of relationships; the exchange of goods is itself merely the tangible means to that goal, an end not well served in the realm of commerce and contract (Murray 1987).

Understanding the significance of gifts among intimates or among small groups such as the Trobrianders or Kwakiutl may leave us puzzled as to what role gifts may play in contemporary society. Hyde ([1925] 1967, 89) wrote:

> Gift exchange is an economy of small groups. . . . It remains an unsolved dilemma of the modern world . . . as to how we are to preserve true community in a mass society, one whose dominant value is exchange value and whose morality has been codified into law.

It would be difficult even to say what "true community" would mean when we are describing not a grouping of a few tribes with a few hundred members each but the multiple, overlapping, and ever-larger and encompassing communities within which we live.

I reside with my family on a street of approximately thirty houses, in a neighborhood and elementary school district of roughly 6,000 people, in a city of 30,000 on the eastern edge of Cleveland, Ohio. The boundaries of my city are indistinct, so that one political entity blends imperceptibly to the next and so on into the city of Cleveland itself or out to the farm country further east.

Which is *the* community? My neighborhood, city, area, county, state, nation, species? We also make communities in other ways, not just by geography. There are communities of scholars and craftsmen, of people with shared political or artistic or culinary interests. Each of these forms of community must solve a related pair of problems: how to ensure that the inevitable occasions for conflict do not sunder the bonds that hold members together; and how to decide what the scope and limits are of the members' obligations to each other, not merely to avoid harm but to render assistance.

At all levels of community, even in my own neighborhood, most of the people are strangers to each other. In the tradition of Western political thought, we are familiar with the idea that we ought not to harm strangers, and that the state may legitimately intervene when others may be harmed through our actions, negligence, or failure to keep our promises. This affords some control over the otherwise terrible threat of boundless conflict. But it does not build community, not in the sense of bonds felt among persons, of solidarity, of standing together in the face of obstacles, natural or human-made.

Community in this sense is desirable even in mass society. At a minimum, it is necessary to support the social structures that permit decent lives to be imagined and shaped. It is necessary to inspire the trust that, if misfortune should strike, individuals will not be abandoned. The dissolution of structures supporting community among the economically and socially dislocated Ik people and the destruction of loyalty and compassion that followed are one illustration of how important community is (Turnbull 1972). Kai Erikson's (1976) study of the loss of community after the Buffalo Creek flood that pushed people back into disorder, fatalism, and dependency is another. People desire community; indeed, they desire it enough to provide for the needs of strangers. Sometimes that provision comes as a result of communal decisions and takes the form of state-enforced provisions—for example, sustaining welfare by redistributing wealth through taxation. Sometimes, though, we prefer to provide for these needs by a system of gifts: It may be gifts of money to individuals or organizations. (Indeed, as a political community we encourage such giving through our tax code.) Or, in the case of the most dramatic gifts to strangers, it may be parts of our own bodies: blood, marrow, even organs.

Published nearly twenty years ago, Richard Titmuss's (1971) *The Gift Relationship: From Human Blood to Social Policy* analyzed the blood-donor systems used in several countries in terms of each culture's values and presumptions. Recognizing the complex motives of individuals who supplied blood, Titmuss nonetheless categorized donors along a rough scale from pure self-interest—the "paid donor"—through a middle ground of mixed and ambiguous motives, to his ideal, the "voluntary community donor," for whom donations are characterized by "the absence of tangible immediate rewards in monetary or nonmonetary forms; the absence of penalties, financial or otherwise; and the knowledge among donors that their donations are for unnamed strangers without distinction of age, sex, medical condition, income, class, religion or ethnic group."

As interesting as his discussion of donors and their motives is Titmuss's (1971, 95) unflattering comparison between the United States, England, and Wales in the mid-1960s. According to his calculations, one-third of all whole blood was purchased outright, more than one-half was tied to replacement or blood insurance schemes, and 5 percent came from a group he dubbed "captive voluntary donors"—prisoners or members of the military. Only 9 percent "approximated to the concept of the voluntary community donor who sees his donation as a free gift to strangers in society." In contrast, almost all blood in England and Wales came from volunteers.

In Titmuss's view, matters in the United States were not only bad, but getting worse, with increasing commercialization of blood. He claimed that "proportionately more blood is being supplied by the poor, the unskilled, the unemployed, Negroes and other low-income groups" and warned that "a new class is emerging of an exploited human population of high blood yielders. Redistribution . . . from the poor to the rich appears to be one of the dominant effects of the American blood banking systems." Another effect of the reliance on donors other than true volunteers was a more dangerous blood supply. Evidence suggested that blood from paid donors was much more likely to cause hepatitis, for example.

Titmuss's analysis was powerful, influential, and—in the matter of

the attitude in the United States toward and reliance on paid donors—mistaken. Contrary to Titmuss's baleful prediction, the United States was moving toward a predominantly volunteer system. By 1982, 70 percent of whole blood was supplied by volunteers, one-quarter through quasi-voluntary "blood credit" or "blood insurance" programs and no more than 3 or 4 percent by paid donors. The proportion of paid donors was declining.

When residents of the United States were asked about blood they overwhelmingly favored a voluntary system and rejected the purchase of blood; when American blood donors were asked why they gave, the typical answer was simply that it was needed. The authors of *The American Blood Supply* summarize their findings thus:

> All our own experiences lead us to believe that participation in the whole-blood supply is the natural, unforced response of a great many people once they are exposed to a mild degree of personal solicitation and some convenient donation opportunities (Drake, Finkelstein, and Sapolsky 1982).

Where communities could not meet their own needs for blood, the explanation typically lay in rivalry or incompetence.

If Titmuss misjudged the generosity of the American people, he was only guilty of the same error as those who set up the system. When Titmuss looked, he found a blood-supply system predicated on the belief that Americans would only part with their blood if there was something in it for them, or at least for those close to them such as family members. In fact, much like their English and Welsh counterparts, Americans needed only to be shown that blood was needed to make them feel that they ought to give it. This point is worth stressing because it is central to the argument: People require no further reason and no other motivation to give blood than to be persuaded that blood is, in fact, needed by others.

Titmuss asked a sample of British donors why they gave. Many of them invoked in one way or another the needs of others. One young woman wrote (with original spelling preserved):

> You cant get blood from supermarkets and chaine stores. People them selves must come forword, sick people cant get out of bed to ask you for a pint to save thier life so I came forword in hope to help somebody who needs blood.

Others wrote of gratitude or reciprocity: "Because I have enjoyed good health all my life and in a small way it is a way of saying 'Thank you' and a small donation to the less fortunate"; "To try and repay in some small way some unknown person whose blood helped me recover from two operations and enable me to be with my family"; "Some unknown person gave blood to save my wife's life." Some put it in terms of duty, or wanting to assure that blood was available should they or someone they loved need it. One middle-aged man gave a brief but eloquent explanation of why he began to give: "1941. War. Blood needed. I had some. Why not?" Or as one worker who had donated 19 times put it: "No money to spare. Plenty of blood to spare."

The distinguished economist Kenneth Arrow (1972) found all this puzzling. He called it "impersonal altruism" and said it was "as far removed from the feelings of personal interaction as any marketplace." Unable to find in the model of self-interested, rational, satisfaction-maximizing economic man the mundane human motivation that would inspire such apparently nonself-interested behavior, he described British donors as "an aristocracy of saints" and ascribed the phenomenon to the tradition of Fabian socialism. He doubts, not surprisingly, that a system relying on volunteers could work elsewhere. He was wrong.

There is an interpretation that fits the facts much better. The needs of others—even strangers—tug at us. We often do not think of them; we may avoid being made aware of them. But once we perceive those needs, we experience them as having a moral force. Needs *should* be met; somehow we know that. If we do meet them, we feel good; if we are derelict, we may feel a vague unease. We are not, cannot be, obliged to satisfy personally *every* need of all persons. But we sense that as members of a community we have some responsibility for assuring that other members do not suffer or perish because their needs were unmet.

This interpretation does not presume that people are saintly, or that they act out of an unearthly, pure altruism. Indeed, the historian Michael Ignatieff (1984) may be right when he says: "We need justice, we need liberty, and we need as much solidarity as can be reconciled with justice and liberty." Solidarity, the sense of connectedness with the strangers among whom we live, may be as essential to human flourishing as the need for blood is for human life.

The system of gifts of blood—gifts to strangers—meets the needs of those strangers and in so doing meets the need of all in belonging to, at least, a minimally decent human community, one that expresses concern for the needs of others.

Though good scientific data are lacking, the belief is widely held that certain groups are less likely to give blood, for example, African-Americans. If genuine, such differences could be interpreted as evidence that individuals in those groups do not feel ties to the larger community that would motivate them to donate. One study found blacks in the Washington, D.C. area reluctant to become organ donors for five reasons: lack of awareness about transplants; religious and other beliefs; distrust of the medical community; fears that donors would be declared dead prematurely; and a preference for giving organs and tissues to other blacks (Callender 1987). Another study suggests that the differences have as much to do with social status as with race. Comparing blacks who had not given blood with blacks and whites who had, the researchers found that nondonors were more likely to be poor, less likely to have education beyond high school, and less likely to have received information about or to have been asked to participate in blood donation (Bayton, Jennings, and Callender 1989).

The nature of social connectedness is clarified, then, when the gift is blood. For many cultures blood represents life itself. Blood is also kinship; we have blood relatives; blood is thicker than water. When we wish to affirm a relationship we can share a blood brotherhood. Or if we want to dampen antagonism among families or nations, we can arrange a marriage between members of the two warring parties; the offspring of such unions share blood from both factions. We sometimes describe conflict by saying that bad blood exists between the opponents.

If blood binds and affirms community, then shared blood is a threat when a sense of community is denied. States such as Arkansas and Louisiana have in the past had laws that required labeling blood by "racial" source. In 1967 the South African Institute for Medical Research paid "Bantus, Coloured, and Asians" one rand and "White" suppliers four rands per unit (Titmuss 1971, 191).

The Poisoned Gift

When a gift is given we assume the gift is good. There is no warning comparable to "caveat emptor" in the realm of gifts. In a commercial interaction, we know to be careful because what the other wants is not you or your affection but the thing you are providing: money, an object, a service. We must be vigilant to ensure that what we receive is what we are promised, that it is not shoddy or dangerous. The usual purpose of a gift is to initiate or affirm a relationship, not to transfer property. If we are wary of entering into a relationship with the giver, or suspect that his/her motives may have more to do with manipulation and control than mutuality, we have reason to be apprehensive about the giver's motives, but even then not about the gift itself. Only a very foolish person gives a shabby gift. Only a very wicked person knowingly gives a gift that harms: a poisoned gift.

The idea of a poisoned gift is an old one. The German word "gift," which comes from the same root as our Anglo-Saxon one, means "poison." The theme of the poisoned gift appears in folk tales as a grave evil. Probably the best-known one is the Grimms' tale "Little Snow White." The Queen, disguised as an old woman, offers Snow White an apple, which she refuses:

> "Are you afraid of poison?" said the old woman; "look, I will cut the apple in two pieces; you eat the red cheek, and I will eat the white." The apple was so cunningly made that only the red cheek was poisoned. Snow-white longed for the fine apple, and when she saw that the woman ate part of it she could resist no longer, and stretched out her hand and took the poisonous half. But hardly had she a bit of it in her mouth than she fell down dead (Eliot 1937).

Contriving to use a gift to harm another is especially chilling because gift exchange presumes that one desires — for whatever reason — to please the other. We may be wary of the giver's reasons for pursuing a relationship with us, but, except for gifts from enemies (and the possibility they may be Trojan horses), we are not accustomed to being suspicious of the gift itself.

Recall the horror years ago when it first became known that some people were giving poisoned gifts to masked (not faceless) victims: Halloween trick-or-treaters. The victims were children; the occasion (whatever its origins), now a celebration. Our horror was comprised of indivisible portions: horror at the innocence and youth of the victims; the violation of the occasion; the harm done to neighbors and strangers; and, finally, that the evil was disguised as a gift.

With AIDS came awareness that the gift of blood itself could be poisoned. With that awareness came a double threat to the community's sense of its own wholeness as some groups were seen to be making not merely poisonous gifts, but poisonous gifts of that which historically has been a fluid of social cohesion. Gifts build relationships. Blood affirms relationship. Gifts of blood confirm our relationship with the strangers with whom we live and share blood, metaphorically and, through our donations, literally. Poisoned blood, when the sources can be identified with particular groups, transforms a solidarity-building practice into a sharp instrument of division and difference.

When blood was recognized as a vector for AIDS, and when gay men, IV drug users, and certain immigrant groups were identified as principal sources of HIV-contaminated blood, the bonds of community were threatened. To many people, men who had sex with other men, people who used drugs, and foreigners—especially dark-skinned foreigners—were already different. The distance from "different" to "dangerous" is short. It was a distance easily covered once the nature of the danger to the blood supply became known.

To people already suspicious and fearful of gay men and others in "high-risk groups," the idea that they were now imperiled by infectious blood must have weakened whatever tenuous communal links they felt for those donors. One important means of affirming community with strangers was transformed suddenly into testimony to the alienism and peril posed by certain of those strangers. There were two crises. First, we had to minimize the danger to those who needed blood or blood products. This was accomplished with remarkable speed. The second crisis was more subtle and less tractable.

It was important to protect the imperiled bonds of community with those now perceived as potentially threatening. Those bonds needed protection lest individuals identified with those groups come to be seen ultimately as "others"—not merely strangers but those who no longer belong to my community. This would be disastrous not only for those who would now be placed in a kind of internal ostracism, but also for the larger community and its members. The gay community recognized well what was at stake:

Just as the threat to blood—symbolic of life itself—galvanized communal anxiety, the threat of exclusion from the blood donor pool represented a profound threat to the social standing of those who would be classed as a danger to the public health. . . . The debate over the blood supply thus placed into question the gay struggle for social integration (Bayer 1989, 73).

According to Ronald Bayer's account of events, leaders in the gay community responded on two fronts. To the rest of the world, including blood bankers and public officials, they presented a list of "do nots": Do not cast us as the villains who infect others; do not treat us as a homogeneous group; do not make or keep lists of our names; do not ask prospective donors questions about sexual orientation or practices. To the members of the gay community, leaders, especially physicians, counseled restraint.

The first likely cases of AIDS caused by blood or blood products were reported in July 1982. By August a gay physician was warning promiscuous gay men not to give blood until more was known. By December of that year, transfusions had been tentatively linked to AIDS as well. In that same month, James Curran, chief of the Centers for Disease Control AIDS efforts, urged the gay community to seize the initiative by calling for gays to refrain from giving blood. At the same time that gay activists were comparing calls by nongays not to give blood to racism and the internment of Japanese-Americans during World War II, and warning against the divisiveness of singling out particular groups as sources of infected blood, they were urging self-restraint within the gay community. A statement by over 50 gay organizations put it thus in January 1983: "In giving the 'gift of life' there is the responsibility to give the safest gift possible" (Bayer 1989, 81).

Most HIV infections occurred in the interval between when the virus first appeared in this country and the adoption of measures to reduce the chance of using infected blood. In March 1983 the U.S. Public Health Service (1983) recommended that members of groups at increased risk for AIDS should refrain from donating blood. The major agencies concerned with the blood supply followed within days with a promise to comply with these recommendations, adopt uniform procedures, and seek the cooperation of the groups at risk. In March 1985, a screening test (the now familiar enzyme-linked immunosorbent assay [ELISA]) was licensed for screening blood donors for antibodies to the virus. It is estimated today that the risk of HIV infection through blood or blood products is between 1 in 100,000 and 200,000. New cases of blood-related AIDS will continue to occur, however, in the pool of already-infected persons who have not yet shown symptoms of AIDS. But the number of new transfusion-related AIDS cases will decline, as will the proportion of AIDS cases caused by transfusions of blood or blood products. Even the sources of clotting factors have changed, moving away from preparation methods that pooled thousands or even tens of thousands of donors to methods that involve a few. We now have the prospect of producing them with cloned genes inserted into microbes, avoiding any possibility of viral contamination.

Ironically, one result of AIDS may be fewer deaths and injuries caused by tainted blood. Transfusion has never been a perfectly safe procedure. In addition to the reactions caused by immune incompatibilities, blood can carry a variety of infectious organisms — most notably, those that cause hepatitis. Prior to AIDS, many patients *and* physicians had too casual an attitude toward blood. Homologous transfusions were used more often than necessary. As well as putting an end to the casual use of transfusions, AIDS also led to the wider use of other existing techniques for replacing or recovering blood lost during surgery. Blood bankers had long encouraged people whose need for blood is predictable — true for much elective surgery — to have blood taken and stored in advance for reinfusion in surgery: autologous ("self") transfusion. Autologous transfusions eliminate the possibility of receiving incompatible blood or blood carrying new infectious agents. Similarly, techniques are available to recover and reinfuse the patient's own blood during surgery (called "intra-operative salvage").

In addition to the awareness of the risks of homologous blood transfusion, increased screening and testing have made the blood used in necessary transfusions much safer. Donors are screened more carefully, and more are "deferred" — a blood bank euphemism for rejection. Blood is now tested routinely for: ABO and Rh type; red-cell-related antibodies (from previous transfusion or pregnancy); syphilis; HIV antibodies; HTLV-I antibodies; Hepatitis B; and a marker for Hepatitis C. A test for antibodies to Hepatitis C will soon be added. The environment in which decisions to adopt new tests are made seems to have changed as a consequence of AIDS, now inclining toward using any test that *might* be beneficial, even though many may have doubts about whether a particular test is worthwhile. An example of that is the new test for HTLV-I, a rare virus that causes cancer in some people. One blood-bank official estimates that it will add $2.80 to the direct cost of each unit of blood, with additional monies spent on confirmatory tests, counseling, and tracing (Barnes 1988).

The experience of donating blood has changed as well. In 1979 you would have taken five minutes to give a health history. The most sensitive question asked on it was whether or not you had ever injected drugs. You were asked if you had ever had or been exposed to hepatitis, or if you had ever turned yellow (hepatitis again), or had a recent cold or flu. If the interview stations had to be crammed together, threatening privacy, no one cared. A finger stick was made for a blood count, and you were ready to donate. The whole process took less than an hour. Deferral rates were about 8 to 9 percent. The reasons people were deferred carried no menacing social baggage — a recent cold, a low red-cell count.

Today, when you arrive to give blood at a Red Cross station, you are first handed a pamphlet: *What You Must Know before Giving Blood.* The only other words on the cover (except for the organization's name) say plainly: "If you are a man who has had sex with another man since 1977, you must not give blood or plasma." Inside the leaflet, along with a brief description of what to expect as a donor, is a section titled "Patient Safety." It warns in bold type "Do not give blood if you are at risk for getting and spreading the AIDS virus," and then lists in detail factors placing you at risk. When your health history is taken, you will be asked about injecting drugs (as in 1979) but there are new questions — about AIDS antibody tests; exposure to AIDS; travel to Haiti or Africa since 1977. You are asked to affirm that you read the pamphlet and that if you are at risk, you will not donate. Now, people are more sensitive to confidentiality and are less willing to give their health history if others might overhear. In addition, you will be given a card that repeats the list of risk factors, and instructed to read it and select one of the two peel-and-stick bar codes (that cannot be read by anyone at the collection site): "Transfuse" or "Do Not Transfuse." If your health history and brief examination confirm your fitness to donate, you will go to the donor room where, except for a more thorough confirmation of your identity (name, address, birth date, Social Security number) and the sometimes conspicuous wearing of gloves, your experience will not be different from donors of ten years ago. The process now takes an hour and one-quarter — all of the added time in screening prior to donation. Because of additional precautions, more donors are deferred (10 to 11 percent in the Cleveland area). Deferral has come to have a different meaning. Individuals who are deferred are likely to feel hurt, rejected—or fearful that they may have AIDS. If you have come with a group to donate, the others may attach onerous significance to your being deferred.

The donation experience has also changed for the professionals and volunteers who staff the stations. The story of the gloves is as good a way to describe this as any. On the day before Thanksgiving 1987, a new rule ordered everyone who came in contact with blood to wear gloves. At a typical blood-collection station this included the interviewers (who did finger sticks), the volunteers who carried the filled bags of blood, the phlebotomists—just about everyone. With the job getting more complicated and with fears about possible risks of infection, fewer volunteers came forward. (One effect of this is that blood centers have had to hire more paid staff, further raising the cost of blood.) Some donors were insulted that everyone was wearing gloves, as if they—the donors—were untouchables. In June 1988 the rule was relaxed. Gloves must now be worn only in a few circumstances, although one may choose to wear them at other times.

AIDS has provoked many changes in the collection and transfusion of blood. Some of the changes are clearly for the better: more cautious use of blood; more use of alternative ways of meeting an individuals's need for blood; improvements in screening donors and testing blood. Some changes, though, have a mixed benefit because we choose to err on the side of not allowing possibly infected blood to be transfused. Thus, while more intensive screening of donors has probably prevented some transmission of blood-borne diseases, it has also resulted in the acceptance of many "false positives"—test results suggesting the presence of virus when the blood is actually safe, thereby irritating, frightening, and possibly stigmatizing, many healthy, uninfectious donors. And some changes are undesirable: large numbers of persons find that their blood is unwanted, including gay men and immigrants from Haiti and Africa. Others fear possible rejection and do not volunteer to donate at all.

A study by Edward H. Kaplan and Alvin Novick estimates that self-deferral between April 1983 and April 1985 prevented between 44 and 52 percent of the possible transfusion-related transmissions of HIV. They estimate the number of averted infections conservatively at between 2,260 and 2,700 (Kaplan and Novick 1989).

Public health officials and blood bankers were moving at a roughly similar pace. In January 1983 the three main blood-banking organizations called for education and voluntary self-deferral, and rejected questions about sexual orientation or practices. As evidence of infection in gay men and transmission through blood grew, explicit warnings were introduced.

The impact of the loss of gay men as potential donors on the blood supply has been difficult to judge. Among blood bankers, gay men were thought to be people who were very willing to donate. Evidence from San Francisco and New York City, though, finds no evidence that gay men were more likely to be donors than other people prior to 1983. AIDS did have a dramatic impact on the blood supply in some locales. Between December 1982 and December 1983, blood donations in San Francisco dropped 20 percent. (Blood use also dropped 20 percent, so a shortage was averted.) Dr. Herbert Perkins (personal communication), director of the Irwin Memorial Blood Centers there, attributes the drop both to the loss of gay males as potential donors and to the widespread misconception that one can get AIDS by donating blood.

At the San Francisco blood bank, autologous donations, which once constituted less than 1 percent of all donated blood, now comprise 5 to 7 percent. Directed donations (i.e., blood donation by an individual for another identified individual), which that bank agreed to do in June 1984, account for roughly the same percentage. Directed donation, touted by proponents as safe, had been resisted by blood banks for several reasons, among them the claim that blood from identified donors might be less safe than blood from anonymous donors. Irwin Memorial's experience is that the risk of HIV infection from directed donations is the same as that from anonymous donors — in both cases extremely small. Directed donors are, however, more likely to have positive tests for hepatitis.

For a time and in some locales, gay women were also rejected as donors (see, e.g., Downton 1986). This is now seen as utterly silly, since gay women have the lowest prevalence of HIV infection of any sexually active group. Blood-bank directors in both New York and San Francisco report that gay women have emerged as organized donor groups for the community and for people with HIV infection in particular; one of the many ironies of AIDS is that those who suffer from it or its precursors are likely themselves to need blood, or at least red-cell transfusions. Gay men support these efforts with their time and effort, though not their blood.

The risk of exclusion, of being perceived as dangerous and cast out, greatly concerned leaders in the gay community. But there was a parallel threat, the mirror image of the broader community's perceptions and actions. Those whose blood was now unacceptable were given the message: "If my gift is to be rejected as dangerous, then I am unworthy to be a giver." Gay men and others with risk factors are thus asked not to participate in this community-affirming practice. Does this mean that they are to be excluded from community in other ways? There are, in fact, many people who are considered unsuitable to give blood. Many of the reasons donors are deferred are temporary: an acute infection, a cold, recent dental work, pregnancy. Other reasons may be cause for permanent deferment: chronic infections such as hepatitis, certain medications that must be taken indefinitely, a history of cancer. People with risk factors for HIV infection are not alone in being advised not to donate blood.

There are other ways to build and affirm community, ways that may lack the symbolic richness of blood but that minister to the needs of strangers. Those at risk of AIDS have a wide range of contributions still open to them. There are still urgent needs for time, effort, and money. Volunteer work, fund raising for community projects that respond to needs otherwise unfulfilled, these and other ways of ministering to the community are all available to gay men as much as to others. Blood remains a powerful way of affirming community, and of contributing to the needs of strangers, but it is not the only way.

AIDS threatens not merely the safety of those who need blood. It also endangers our sometimes fragile bonds of community, those ties that link us to the strangers with whom we live in a mass society. When a particular group of strangers, a group already regarded with some suspicion, comes to be seen as posing a threat to all through their poisonous gifts of blood, we face, I believe, a genuine crisis, one that could weaken further or even sever the bond between that group and the larger community. A number of leaders in the gay community, even as they voiced concerns over possible discrimination, insisted on the need to act responsibly to protect the health of others. And public health leaders, attentive to the history of discrimination and the ripeness of the situation for worsening discrimination, have acted in a measured but firm manner to minimize the danger to health.

Some analysts point out that plasma (the fluid part of blood), and the products obtained from it, tell a different story from the one recounted thus far. Alongside the voluntary, not-for-profit network that obtains whole blood is a proprietary plasma industry that pays its suppliers and seeks profits. Plasmapheresis is a process that separates the blood's liquid and the proteins it contains from the red and white cells, which are then returned to the body. An individual can sell plasma as often as once a week at $10 to $15 a unit. The plasma is then used by pharmaceutical companies to manufacture a variety of products. Plasma products have transmitted HIV, just as whole blood has.

The plasmapheresis industry is just that—an industry. Suppliers are mistakenly called "donors," but that use is parasitic on genuine blood donation and should be abandoned. There is no gift given here; the transaction is clearly commercial. In 1985 the U.S. Congress Office of Technology Assessment predicted the demise of commercial plasmapheresis:

> By the end of the century, there is a real chance that plasma as a source of current biological proteins will be replaced by recombinant DNA and monoclonal antibody technologies . . . the longstanding controversy over commercial plasma donors may be solved, not through implementation of a deliberate, contested public policy, but through advances in technology which could make the voluntary v. commercial policy debate moot (1985, 37).

Applied researchers are already at work on the manufacture of biological proteins that plasma now supplies. A biosynthetic version of one such protein, clotting Factor VIII, has been in clinical trials for three years; biosynthetic albumin is available, but not economically competitive with albumin derived from plasma.

Some U.S. blood banks have begun their own noncommercial plasmapheresis programs similar to ones in Canada and other countries, which do not rely on a commercial plasmapheresis system. Voluntary programs in this country may grow even more with the recent invention of an automated plasmapheresis machine that is safer and faster than earlier processes. With the new device, giving a unit of plasma takes only about ten minutes longer than donating a unit of whole blood. As far as donors are concerned, the current difference between plasmapheresis and whole-blood donation may one day largely disappear.

Some voices, furthermore, have called for the recommodification of whole blood, a measure that in effect runs counter to the social solidarity that voluntary donations engender. Harvey M. Sapolsky (1989, 146) recently suggested that the safety of transfusions be enhanced by means that "require the breaking of this bond of community, improving chances for some recipients while perhaps harming those of others." He names three strategies: directed donation, obtaining blood from regions with a low incidence of HIV infection, and paying donors from presumably low-risk groups. Sapolsky (1989, 158) appears to be no admirer of not-for-profit blood banks: "Protecting organizations that hold small empires and convenient ideologies does not reduce the risk of transfusion or build community." One need not believe that blood banks are perfectly virtuous to find Sapolsky's attack overwrought and his solution misguided.

The most thorough estimate of the current risk of HIV in the blood supply (Cumming et al. 1989) indicates that the risk, while present, is small and declining: the number of undetected HIV-positive units in 1987 is 131 — one unit in every 153,123. The rate of infected blood has been dropping by 30 percent a year. A preliminary analysis of the data for 1988 shows a further drop of 34 percent to 87 units. The improvement is likely due to a combination of factors: better education and self-deferral, more donors who are repeatedly HIV negative.

It is not clear that the measures Sapolsky proposes would be an improvement over what blood banks have been doing. Sapolsky's call for more directed donations is unlikely to lead to safer blood. Blood banks have not been enthusiastic about directed blood donations. Even proponents of directed donations admit that they significantly increase administrative complexity and costs (Goldfinger 1989). In theory the advantage of directed donations is that you know who the donors are and what exposures they might have had. This supposed advantage is offset by other considerations. Directed donors are more likely to be first-time donors, and first-time donors are more likely to have previously undetected diseases. Because their identity is known, directed donors might be less willing to admit to risk factors lest they suffer disapproval from family and friends. The evidence on the relative safety of directed versus homologous donations shows no significant difference thus far (Page 1989). In certain types of directed donations, for example, parents donating to their newborn infants, there may be added risks because of subtle, undetected incompatibilities with consequences as severe as graft-versus-host disease (Strauss et al. 1990). One potential advantge of directed donor programs is that they could allow individuals who need multiple transfusions to receive them from the same few donors, resulting in less stress to the immune system (Strauss et al. 1990). Autologous blood remains the safest method; a study of elective surgery patients found that those storing directed donations along with autologous blood were no less likely to need additional homologous blood than those relying solely on autologous transfusions (Goodnough 1989). Except in unusual circumstances, directed donation appears to be more expensive but no safer than homologous blood. The case for "breaking . . . this bond of community" in order to improve transfusion safety is weak at best. Directed donations are as likely to add HIV-positive units to the blood supply as they are to subtract from them.

Paying donors to encourage "safer" populations, such as women or middle-aged people, is unnecessary. Blood banks have recently directed their efforts toward safer donor populations with considerable success. Sapolsky's other suggestion — obtaining more blood from communities with low incidence of HIV infection — does not necessarily break any bonds of community. It could just as well be seen as a way of expanding the scope of community.

AIDS poses a continuing threat to the blood supply, in the form of lawsuits against blood banks on behalf of people who allege that they were infected with HIV through blood or blood products. Blood banks fear that multimillion-dollar judgments, awarded by a few juries thus far, could disrupt severely their operations, even forcing some into bankruptcy. Agencies will not reveal the number of pending suits, but a figure of 200 to 300 has been reported (Blakeslee 1989).

There are two critical periods in the control of AIDS pertinent to the suits against blood banks. The first was the accumulation of evidence that AIDS was indeed a blood-borne disease, beginning in late 1982, gathering strength in 1983, and culminating in the discovery of the virus in 1984. In hindsight it may be difficult to remember the several competing theories about what causes AIDS, a number of which remained plausible well into 1983. The March 1983 recommendation by the CDC that donors engaging in high-risk behaviors defer themselves suggested a standard of conduct for blood banks that they rapidly adopted. The second critical period came in the spring of 1985, with the licensing of the ELISA test. Blood banks that did not quickly adopt self-deferral programs in 1983 or ELISA screening in 1985 are vulnerable to charges that they behaved negligently. Some heart-rending suits allege that the individual was infected by blood collected the day before ELISA testing began (Blakeslee 1989).

Current law in most states classifies blood as a "service" rather than a "product." If blood were a product being sold, then the seller could be held strictly liable for damage caused by it if the conditions for imposing strict liability, including "unreasonable dangerousness," are met (Hall 1989). Otherwise the injured party would have to prove that the blood bank acted negligently, or failed in its duty to warn of the risks of blood transfusion or to inform about alternatives to homologous donations such as autologous or directed donation (Gostin 1990). Fear of future litigation is probably among the factors prompting blood banks to adopt new screening tests and other procedures. The community's needs, that is, will be met, but at increased expense, some exasperation on the part of those who believed they were doing a service, and alienation and anger from those who were hurt.

I have written much about community here, about our need for it, and about how the community provision of blood to those who need it acknowledges and reinforces the ties we have even to the strangers among whom we live. Biological needs like blood are part of a language of need that all can understand. But there are forces pulling us apart as well. Ignatieff describes the conflict: "The centripetal forces of need, labour and science which are pulling us together as a species are counter-balanced by centrifugal forces, the claims of tribe, race, class, section, region and nation, pulling us apart" (1984, 130–31). Blood, like anything else, can be used—has been used—to divide as well as to bind. The poor and the disfavored may look with suspicion at requests that they donate to a community they feel may have treated them unfairly. Communities who believe their blood is safer may try to keep it for themselves, just as in the past some communities tried to separate "white" blood from "black" (as if it were not all red).

Blood alone will not magically solve the problem modernity poses— how to keep the language and the practice of solidarity alive in an era when our mobility and communications blur the distinction between neighbor and stranger. We can witness the calamities befalling people half a planet away or listen to strangers reveal intimate secrets, perhaps while family members sit silently nearby. Ignatieff reminds us of our own ingenuity, how the nineteenth-century city, for example, invented: "the boulevard, the public park, the museum, the café, the trolley car, street lighting, the subway, the railway, the apartment house. Each of these humble institutions created a new possibility for fraternity among strangers in public places" (1984, 140). Our century has surely invented more, not least of which is the blood bank.

Those who understood the moral issues at stake, articulated them, and insisted public policy be based on them, helped avert what could have been a lasting blow to the effort to enlarge our collective sense of community. Blood banking has changed significantly. Health professionals and the public now understand better that for all its life-giving properties, blood can also be harmful. But people still donate by the million. And countless lives are saved by donated blood. AIDS does not appear to have altered in any fundamental way the meaning of gifts of blood for giver or recipient.

Human need continues to take many forms. The recent earthquake in the Bay area reminds us of that. On the day after the quake, 649 people stood in line for as much as four hours to give blood at the San Francisco blood bank. This was ten times the normal number for a weekday. Dr. Herbert Perkins (personal communication) says that they came for two reasons: because victims of the quake were in need, and the donors wanted to do something to help; and because they wanted company in this chaotic time. That is, they responded to need in the community at the same time as they demonstrated their own need for community. As long as we need solidarity, and members of our community have needs, there will be a place for gifts, such as blood, that affirm community by ministering to need.

References

American Red Cross. 1988. *What You Must Know before Giving Blood.* Washington.

Arrow, K.J. 1972. Gifts and Exchanges. *Philosophy and Public Affairs* 1(4):355–60.

Barnes, D.M. 1988. HTLV-I: To Test or Not to Test. *Science* 242:372–73.

Bayer, R. 1989. *Private Acts, Social Consequences: AIDS and the Politics of Public Health.* New York: Free Press.

Bayton, J.A., P.S. Jennings, and C.O. Callender. 1989. The Role of Blacks in Blood Donation and the Organ and Tissue Transplantation Process. *Transplantation Proceedings* 21(6):3971–72.

Blackstone, W. 1765–1769. *Commentaries on the Laws of England.* London.

Blakeslee, S. 1989. Blood Banks Facing Hundreds of AIDS Suits. *New York Times* (April 27):B19.

Callender, C.O. 1987. Organ Donation in Blacks: A Community Approach. *Transplantation Proceedings* 19(1):1551–54.

Centers for Disease Control. 1990. *HIV/AIDS Surveillance*. February. Atlanta.

Cumming, P.D., E.L. Wallace, J.B. Schorr, and R.Y. Dodd. 1989. Exposure of Patients to Human Immunodeficiency Virus through the Transfusion of Blood Components That Test Antibody Negative. *New England Journal of Medicine* 321(14):941–46.

Downton, J.H. 1986. Should Lesbians Give Blood? *Lancet* 2 (August 16):398.

Drake, A.W., S.N. Finkelstein, and H.M. Sapolsky. 1982. *The American Blood Supply*. Cambridge: MIT Press.

Eliot, C.W. 1937. *Folk-Lore and Fable: Aesop, Grimm, Andersen*. New York: Collier.

Emerson, R.E. [1844] 1979. Gifts, in *Essays of Ralph Waldo Emerson*. Norwalk, CT: Easton.

Erikson, K.T. 1976. *Everything In Its Path: Destruction of Community in the Buffalo Creek Flood*. New York: Simon and Schuster.

Goldfinger, D. 1989. Directed Blood Donations: Pro. *Transfusion* 29(1):70–74.

Goodnough, L.T. 1989. Directed Blood Procurement Does Not Benefit Patients Who Are Enrolled in an Autologous Blood Predeposit Program. *American Journal of Clinical Pathology* 92(4):484–87.

Gostin, L.O. 1990. The AIDS Litigation Project: A National Review of Court and Human Rights Commission Decisions. Part I: The Social Impact of AIDS. *Journal of the American Medical Association* 263(14):1961–70.

Hall, T.S. 1989. Bad Blood: Blood Industry's Immunity from Liability for Transfusion-borne Disease. *Journal of Products Liability* (12):25–44.

Hyde, L. 1983. *The Gift: Imagination and the Erotic Life of Property*. New York: Vintage.

Ignatieff, M. 1984. *The Needs of Strangers: An Essay on Privacy, Solidarity, and the Politics of Being Human*. New York: Viking.

Kaplan, E.H., and A. Novick. 1989. Self-deferral, HIV Infection, and the Blood Supply. New Haven: Yale University, School of Organization and Management (Kaplan), or Department of Biology (Novick). (Unpublished.)

Mauss, M. [1925] 1967. *The Gift: Forms and Functions of Exchange in Archaic Societies*. New York: Norton.

Murray, T.H. 1987. Gifts of the Body and the Needs of Strangers. *Hastings Center Report* 17(2):30–38.

Page, P.L. 1989. Controversies in Transfusion Medicine: Directed Blood Donation: Con. *Transfusion* 29(1):65–70.

Sapolsky, H.M. 1989. AIDS, Blood Banking, and the Bonds of Community. *Daedalus* (Summer):145–63.

Strauss, R.G., A. Barnes, Jr., V.S. Blanchette, S.H. Butch, H.A. Hume, G.J. Levy, A. McMican, K. Starling, and A. Mauer. 1990. Committee Report (Pediatric Hemotherapy Committee, American Association of Blood Banks): Directed and Limited-exposure Blood Donations for Infants and Children. *Transfusion* 30(1):68–72.

Titmuss, R.M. 1971. *The Gift Relationship: From Human Blood to Social Policy.* New York: Pantheon.

Turnbull, C.M. 1972. *The Mountain People.* New York: Simon and Schuster.

U.S. Congress. Office of Technology Assessment. 1985. Blood Policy and Technology: Summary. Washington.

U.S. Public Health Service. 1983. Prevention of Acquired Immune Deficiency Syndrome (AIDS): Report of Interagency Recommendations. *Morbidity and Mortality Weekly Reporter* 32:101–3.

Acknowledgments: Thanks are owed to many people: to Louise Keating, Carolyn Kean, and Janice Querin for their patient efforts to describe the changes in blood banking over the past decade; to Bob Rigney and Jane Mesnard for providing information; and to Ronald Bayer for his generous assistance.

AIDS and the Rights of the Individual
Toward a More Sophisticated Understanding of Discrimination

THOMAS B. STODDARD and WALTER RIEMAN

B ETWEEN 1918 AND 1920, IN RESPONSE TO PUBLIC fears over the spread of venereal diseases, especially concern for the health of the soldiers and sailors conscripted to fight in World War I, the government of the United States promoted and paid for the detention of more than 18,000 women suspected of prostitution (Brandt 1985). Under an act of Congress directing the creation of a "civilian quarantine and isolation fund," women were held against their will in state-run "reformatories" until it could be determined that they were not infectious. The government's program, while startling in size, is hardly unique in the history of American public health. When cholera struck New York City in 1832, officials rounded up alcoholics, especially poor Irishmen, in the belief that the illness arose in part from intemperance. During New York City's polio epidemic of 1916, health officials routinely conducted house-to-house searches and forcibly removed and quarantined children thought to have the disease (Risse 1988).

With AIDS the official response has been remarkably different. So far, the few serious proposals for mass quarantines have failed. The most vocal and visible public health officials, including the former surgeon general of the United States, have championed voluntary mea-

241

sures over coercive ones (Koop 1986). They have generally argued for greater compassion for those afflicted, and for heightened legal protections against discrimination. Indeed, the commission appointed by President Reagan to advise him on AIDS made unfair discrimination the centerpiece of its final report (Presidential Commission on the Human Immunodeficiency Virus Epidemic 1988).

What accounts for the turnabout? The answer may lie partly in the nature of the disease. HIV, the virus believed to cause AIDS, is fragile and difficult to transmit. But venereal diseases are also difficult to transmit, and yet concern over their spread led to the largest quarantine in American history.

Another factor may be the vigor of the advocacy on behalf of people with AIDS and others affected by the epidemic. AIDS is the first epidemic to have a corps of political activists arguing regularly for the rights, concerns, and interests of those who are sick or might become sick. But even the best advocacy cannot overcome massive dread, and, if the polls are correct, as many as one-fifth of the American people fear that they might themselves develop AIDS (Blendon and Donelan 1988). Moreover, these polls also show that a substantial portion of the populace – approximately 30 percent – support some form of quarantine for people with HIV in their blood.

The change in approach has major roots, we believe, in the law. Before the 1950s, American law – despite the promises of the Declaration of Independence, the Bill of Rights, and the Civil War amendments to the federal Constitution – gave only weak and unpredictable support to many core principles of individual rights. In the three decades between 1950 and 1980, however, civil liberties and civil rights received greater sustained attention than they had at any time since Reconstruction. In the courts, a long struggle over government-sponsored race discrimination led to the Supreme Court's decision in *Brown v. Board of Education*,[1] which condemned racial segregation in public schools as unconstitutionally denying black Americans equal protection under the law. In other cases decided during this period, the Supreme Court invalidated numerous historically rooted features of law that invidiously favored one group of persons over another. The invalidated legal provisions in-

---

[1] *Brown v. Board of Education*, 347 U.S. 483 (1954).

cluded, for example, the poll tax, traditional methods of drawing boundaries for electoral districts, and various statutes discriminating against women.

Over the same period, state and local legislatures addressed for the first time discrimination by privately owned businesses, and enacted laws forbidding employment decisions based on race, national origin, religion, gender, and other categories. Congress followed suit with the Civil Rights Act of 1964,[2] and one year later acted against racial discrimination in the electoral process through the Voting Rights Act of 1965.[3]

The broad cultural developments that brought about these revolutionary shifts in the law are many: our changed sense of nationhood after World War II, postwar prosperity, the civil rights movement for black Americans, the movement against the war in Vietnam, and the emergence of a newer and more radical feminism. The general thrust of the changes, we believe, is reasonably clear; between 1950 and 1980 American law came to embrace the principle of eliminating prejudice based on factors unrelated to individual merit, and established concrete rules limiting many actions based on bias. This recasting of the law is incomplete; most jurisdictions, for example, still do not prohibit private discrimination on account of a person's marital status or sexual orientation. Nevertheless, the three decades after 1950 did undoubtedly mark a fundamental change in both legal doctrine and cultural values.

AIDS is the first public health crisis to arise after the midcentury civil rights revolution. In this chapter we will consider how this fundamental shift in the law affected society's response to the epidemic. We will also describe how discrimination arising from AIDS highlights the deficiencies and limitations of the Supreme Court's current approach to the constitutional concept of "equal protection of the laws." Finally, we will offer some thoughts on how the epidemic may further transform and refine the law, especially the concept of "equal protection."

---

[2]Civil Rights Act of 1964, Pub. L. 88-352, 78 Stat. 241 (codified as amended at 28 U.S.C. § 1447, 42 U.S.C. §§ 1971, 1975a–1975d, 2000a–2000h-6).
[3]Voting Rights Act of 1965, Pub. L. 89-110, 79 Stat. 241 (codified as amended at 42 U.S.C. § 1973 to 1973bb-4 and notes thereto).

The Development of the American
Statutory Law of Civil Rights
Since World War II

The recent history of the American civil rights movement cannot be told merely by describing the central statutes, executive actions, and judicial decisions in the movement's long struggle. The civil rights movement or movements, since we are concerned with more than the struggle for racial equality, were political in a far more embracing sense — their consequences extended well beyond the law. Nonetheless, legal changes achieved since World War II are among the central features of this revolution in American society. A very brief and necessarily incomplete sketch of how these changes occurred — how the law shifted, or in some instances failed to shift, in ways that promoted equality — is helpful to understanding the law's response to AIDS.

The postwar development of civil rights in this country is the more remarkable in light of the depressing history between Reconstruction and World War II. During Reconstruction, Congress enacted a number of important statutes designed to prohibit racial discrimination by private persons. In 1883, however, the Supreme Court ruled that the fourteenth amendment had not granted Congress the constitutional authority to forbid discrimination by nongovernmental entities.[4] This holding, which survived until 1964, left the problem of racial discrimination by private persons largely to the states.[5]

By 1964, 25 states had enacted laws forbidding racial discrimination in employment (Woll 1964, 94). Thirty-one states and the District of Columbia required places of public accommodation, such as hotels and restaurants, to serve all persons who requested service regardless of race (Caldwell 1965, 842).[6] The federal Civil Rights Act of 1964 extended

---

[4] *Civil Rights Cases*, 109 U.S. 3 (1883).
[5] In 1964 the Supreme Court upheld the power of Congress to forbid racial discrimination by most places of public accommodation: *Heart of Atlanta Motel v. United States*, 379 U.S. 241 (1964). Technically, this case avoided overruling the *Civil Rights Cases* by relying on the power of Congress under the commerce clause. As a practical matter, however, the holding of the *Civil Rights Cases* ceased to have much importance after *Heart of Atlanta Motel*.
[6] S. rep. no. 872, 88th Cong., 2d sess., repr. in *U.S. Code Congressional and Administrative News* 2355 (1964).

similar prohibitions nationwide; it prohibited most private employers and places of public accommodation from discriminating by reason of, among other things, race, color, religion, or national origin. The following year, Congress passed the Voting Rights Act of 1965, which strengthened prohibitions in the Civil Rights Act of 1964 against racial discrimination in the conduct of elections.

The Civil Rights Act of 1964 also prohibited discrimination by most private employers based on sex. This provision had little precedent in state law; in 1964 only three states had legislation barring discrimination based on sex (*Iowa Law Review* 1965). Indeed, the prohibition on sex discrimination in the 1964 act was inserted by opponents of the act in a tactical effort to defeat the entire bill. In 1978 Congress declared that discrimination against "pregnant persons" was unlawful discrimination based on sex.[7] And although the federal Equal Rights Amendment was ratified by only 35 of the necessary 38 states (disregarding purported rescissions of ratification) and therefore failed, by 1977, 17 states had adopted provisions in their state constitutions forbidding sex discrimination by state and local government (Kurtz 1977, 101–2).

In other areas of law related to equality, the states took the lead. For example, by 1966, 23 states had legislatively prohibited age discrimination by private employers (*New York University Law Review* 1966, 388); federal legislation was to follow (Age Discrimination in Employment Act of 1967).[8]

The antidiscrimination statutes that have been most important to people with AIDS or HIV began at the federal level. Only a very few states arguably protected handicapped or disabled people against discrimination when Congress passed the Rehabilitation Act of 1973[9] (*Georgetown Law Journal* 1973, 1502 n.6.). This act prohibits employers that receive federal financial assistance from discriminating against an individual with a "handicapping condition" who is "other-

---

[7]Pregnancy Discrimination Act of 1978, Pub. L. 95-555, 92 Stat. 2076 (amending 42 U.S.C. § 2000e (1982)) (overturning result in *General Electric Co. v. Gilbert*, 429 U.S. 125 (1976)).
[8]Age Discrimination in Employment Act of 1967, Pub. L. 90-202, 81 Stat. 602 (codified as amended at 29 U.S.C. §§ 621-634 and 621 note).
[9]Rehabilitation Act of 1973, Pub. L. 93-112, 87 Stat. 355 (codified as amended at 20 U.S.C. § 1414 note, 29 U.S.C. §§ 701-796i, 701 note, 795m note, 42 U.S.C. § 2000d-7).

wise qualified." In 1987 the Supreme Court held in the case of *School Board of Nassau County v. Arline*[10] that a contagious disease can qualify as a "handicapping condition." Although *Arline* concerned an employee with tuberculosis, the logic of the case compels the conclusion that AIDS is also a "handicapping condition" entitling the affected individual to the protection of the act (Turner 1988). After passage of the federal Rehabilitation Act, the states enacted their own handicap-discrimination laws. Most of those statutes *do* cover private employment, and have been of exceptional assistance to people with AIDS and HIV (Leonard 1989).

When it becomes fully effective in 1992, the Americans with Disabilities Act of 1990[11] will establish a broad federal prohibition against disability-based discrimination by private employers, places of public accommodation, and transportation and communications services. The statute protects asymptomatic persons with HIV infection as well as people with AIDS.[12]

The Supreme Court's Development of the Constitutional Right to Equality

Judicial enforcement of the United States Constitution has also had a critical place in the development of civil rights principles. Starting in the 1950s, the Supreme Court greatly revitalized and strengthened what might be called its jurisprudence of equality. In addition to the Court's race-discrimination cases, that jurisprudence encompasses the constitutional voting-rights cases, which require government to give every citizen's vote equal weight. The Supreme Court's jurisprudence of equality also covers a wide range of freedom of expression and religion cases, which prohibit the majority from violating the right to equality possessed by individuals with unpopular convictions. It extends as well to the Court's criminal procedure decisions, many of which prohibit

---

[10] *School Board v. Arline*, 480 U.S. 273 (1987).
[11] Americans with Disabilities Act of 1990, Pub. L. 101-336, 104 Stat. 327.
[12] E.g., H.R. Rep. no. 485 (II), 101st Cong., 2d sess. 51-52 (1990), repr. in *U.S. Code Congressional and Administrative News* 303, 333–34 (1990); S. Rep. no. 116, 101st Cong., 1st sess. 8, 22 (1989).

government from denying fundamental equality to persons accused of a crime. The government, for example, must advise persons in custody of their rights and provide indigent persons accused of serious crime with free counsel, in part to defend the equality of the uninformed or poor. And finally, the Court's jurisprudence of equality includes the decisions often called privacy cases, to which we will return.

These decisions relied on numerous different constitutional provisions, but many were based on or influenced by the fourteenth amendment to the United States Constitution, which is the primary and most explicit guarantee of equality in the Constitution. That amendment, which was adopted shortly after the Civil War, provides in part that "[no] state shall . . . deny to any person within its jurisdiction the equal protection of the laws." The equal-protection clause, like most other provisions in the United States Constitution, binds only the federal and state governments.[13] The principal purpose of the amendment, however, was to outlaw racial discrimination by the states that had been part of the Confederacy.

Before 1950 the Supreme Court had interpreted the equal-protection clause to provide only very limited rights to equality, even in the area of racial discrimination. Most notoriously, the Court had held that the amendment did not prohibit the states from requiring racial segregation of public facilities, so long as the segregated facilities were "equal."[14] In cases not involving racial discrimination, the force of the amendment was even weaker.

Equal-protection analysis took on a more familiar shape with the modern race-discrimination cases, the most important of which is the 1954 case of *Brown v. Board of Education*. These cases developed the beginnings of what is now frequently called "three-tiered" equal-protection review. Under this scheme, the courts apply three different levels of review in equal-protection cases: "strict scrutiny," "intermediate review," and "rational-basis review."

In *Brown*, a classic "strict-scrutiny" case, the Court held that racially segregated public schools are inherently unequal by reason of, among

---

[13]The equal-protection clause mentions only the states, not the federal government. The Supreme Court has held, however, that actions forbidden to the states by the equal-protection clause are forbidden to the federal government through the due-process clause of the fifth amendment: *Bolling v. Sharpe*, 347 U.S. 497 (1954).

[14]*Plessy v. Ferguson*, 163 U.S. 537 (1896).

other things, the humiliation and insult that racial segregation inevitably inflicts on nonwhite students. The *Brown* opinion emphasized the
importance of public schools in support of its holding, but it soon
came to stand for the broader proposition that racial segregation in any
government-run facility violates the Constitution. Race, the Court determined, is a "suspect" classification, and governmental action based
on race is accordingly subject to "strict scrutiny" under the equal-protection clause. Under the test applied in strict-scrutiny cases, governmental action that discriminates by reason of race is unconstitutional
unless that action is necessary to the achievement of a "compelling" governmental purpose, and unless the action is the narrowest means available
to accomplish that purpose. The Court has also declared governmental
classifications by national origin to be suspect.[15] Setting aside the special case of affirmative action, the courts rarely uphold governmental
conduct disadvantaging the members of a suspect class.

Strict scrutiny also applies to governmental classifications that tres-
pass on certain rights the Court regards as "fundamental." In addition
to rights explicitly protected by other provisions of the Constitution,
the Court has ruled that individuals have a fundamental right to make
certain basic decisions concerning one's body and personal conduct. According to the Court, aspects of this general right are implicit in the
Constitution's guarantees of equal protection under the law and due
process of law, and in certain other constitutional provisions. The cases
identifying aspects of this right, which are often called the privacy
cases, are potentially of great importance in shaping issues of constitutional law that may arise as a result of the AIDS epidemic.

Under the Court's decisions, this right to privacy precludes or sharply
limits governmental interference with personal decisions concerning the
education of one's children;[16] the use of contraception;[17] and—at least
as of this writing—the choice to have an abortion during the early
stages of pregnancy.[18] The Court has largely failed, however, to articulate an overarching theory explaining the scope of these decisions or
even to define the term "privacy." One plausible explanation for the
privacy cases is the general proposition that individuals have a core

---

[15] *Mathews v. Lucas*, 427 U.S. 495, 504 (1976).
[16] *Meyer v. Nebraska*, 262 U.S. 390 (1923).
[17] *Griswold v. Connecticut*, 381 U.S. 479 (1965).
[18] *Roe v. Wade*, 410 U.S. 113 (1973).

right to individual autonomy—to make certain basic personal decisions for themselves, where those decisions will not harm others. Under the privacy cases, severe infringements on the liberty of persons with HIV—for example, quarantine—might well trigger heightened judicial review (Parmet 1986, 84–87).

Recent decisions, however, have rejected constitutional challenges to statutes that criminalize private homosexual conduct among adults[19] and that extensively regulate abortion.[20] These cases call into question whether individuals will retain significant constitutional rights to privacy or autonomy under the new majority of conservative justices on the Court.

In another series of constitutional cases beginning in 1971, the Supreme Court began to treat with hostility governmental discrimination based on gender. The Court has not, however, applied to sex-discrimination cases the same stringent equal-protection standard that governs racial classifications. Legislative classifications by sex, according to the Court, must serve "important" (as opposed to "compelling") governmental objectives and must be "substantially related" (rather than "necessary") to achievement of those objectives.[21] This less demanding form of review is the second equal-protection tier, often referred to as "intermediate review." The Court also subjects governmental action disadvantaging illegitimate children and aliens to "intermediate" review.

The Court does not subject these classifications to strict scrutiny because it evidently regards them as arguably relevant to some limited number of legislative purposes. By contrast, the Court subjects racial classifications to a harsher standard because they are generally irrelevant to *any* appropriate legislative purpose, and because the equal-protection clause was specifically intended to eradicate the historical consequences of slavery.

Finally, the third and least demanding "tier" of equal-protection examination is "rational-basis" review, which merely requires that governmental action be rationally related to a legitimate governmental purpose. This form of review makes only very minimal demands, and, consequently, legislation reviewed under the test nearly always passes

---

[19]*Bowers v. Hardwick*, 478 U.S. 186 (1986).
[20]*Webster v. Reproductive Health Services*, 109 S. Ct. 3040 (1989).
[21]*Craig v. Boren*, 429 U.S. 190 (1976).

muster. It is the catch-all or residual test: all acts of federal, state, and local government that classify individuals—i.e., that treat some individuals differently from others—and are not subject to strict or intermediate scrutiny must be "rational."

The Supreme Court has never explained convincingly why three different equal-protection tests are necessary to interpret the one equal-protection clause in the federal Constitution. But the three-tiered structure would not have survived its critics if it did not serve some purpose that the Court is unwilling to sacrifice. What purpose the Court's rather arcane equal-protection structure, in fact, serves—and why that structure is unhelpful in constructing a theory of equality that is adequate for persons disadvantaged for reasons related to their own or another's actual or perceived HIV status—is illuminated by looking at two cases in which the Court did not apply its usual framework.

The Inadequacy of Current Constitutional Doctrine for Cases Involving HIV

Among the most serious problems with the Court's equal-protection structure is that it requires the Court to apply the *same* level of review to *all* governmental uses of a particular classification, regardless of the use to which the government puts the classification in a particular regulation. Because the government is sometimes but not always justified in treating people with AIDS or HIV differently, this undiscriminating approach to equal protection is poorly suited to equal-protection issues involving them.

In two cases, the Court has seemed to recognize the possibility of a different approach to equal protection. In *Plyler v. Doe*,[22] decided in 1982, the plaintiffs challenged a Texas statute limiting state funding of public education as a violation of the equal-protection clause. Texas granted a free education in the public schools to children who were citizens of the United States or were legally admitted to the United States. The Texas statute attacked in *Plyler* denied, however, a free public education to children who could not prove that they were legally admitted to the United States. Texas argued, in substance, that it had no obligation to spend its money educating children whose very presence in the state was unlawful.

---

[22] *Plyler v. Doe*, 457 U.S. 202 (1982).

Attorneys for the excluded children attacked the Texas statute as unconstitutional under the equal-protection clause. They argued that the excluded children could not be blamed for the misdeeds of their parents. The attorneys also argued that the Texas statute could not realistically be expected to diminish illegal immigration. Instead, the main result of the statute, they claimed, would be to promote the creation of a permanent uneducated underclass in Texas.

The statute attacked in *Plyler* did not deny any right the Court views as "fundamental"; the Court had already ruled in 1973 that there is no fundamental right to public education.[23] Moreover, *Plyler* did not involve discrimination based on a classification that is always or even usually irrelevant to governmental purpose, such as race or sex. A person's status as an undocumented alien is highly relevant to, for example, a deportation proceeding. Thus, the Court was required to consider whether the classification that Texas had used — lack of documentation proving the right to live in the United States — was appropriate in light of the *specific purpose* to which Texas had put that classification.

By a vote of five to four, the Supreme Court ruled that the Texas statute was unconstitutional. The majority observed that the Texas statute "impose[d] a lifetime hardship on a discrete class of children not accountable for their disabling status." This fact, according to the majority, meant that the Texas statute "can hardly be considered rational unless it furthers some substantial goal of the state." The Court found that it furthered no such goal, and consequently held it unconstitutional.

Cleburne v. Cleburne Living Center,[24] which was decided in 1985, three years after *Plyler*, is reminiscent of that case. In *Cleburne*, the city of Cleburne, Texas, denied a private organization's application to build a group home for the mentally retarded in a residential neighborhood. The city claimed that it was acting under a zoning ordinance designed to protect mentally retarded persons from floods, harassment from local school children, overcrowding, and various other alleged hazards in the neighborhood. The Supreme Court, however, found that the mentally retarded did not need any greater protection from such potential harms than the aged, the physically ill, and other persons permitted to live in the neighborhood. The Court concluded that

---

[23]*Rodriguez v. San Antonio Independent School District*, 411 U.S. 1 (1973).
[24]*Cleburne v. Cleburne Living Center*, 473 U.S. 432 (1985).

the city's claimed justifications for the denial of the permit reflected "an irrational prejudice against the mentally retarded." The Court, therefore, found that the city's decision failed even the highly deferential rational-basis test. Consequently, even though the Court stated that the mentally retarded are *not* a suspect class, it held the city's decision to be unconstitutional.

In an important separate opinion, Justice Stevens criticized the entire three-tiered framework. He argued that under the equal-protection clause, governmental classifications should be upheld only if "an impartial lawmaker could logically believe that the classification would serve a legitimate public purpose that transcends the harm to the members of the disadvantaged class." Judged by this unitary standard, he found the city's zoning decision to be unconstitutional.

Plyler and *Cleburne* must be viewed as cases in which the Court was forced to face the inadequacies of its own theories of equal protection. In each, the Court was faced with a morally repugnant denial by the government of equal concern and respect for individuals under its control. And in each, the Court rightly held those denials of equal concern and respect to be unconstitutional. The hard question is not really why the Court decided *Plyler* and *Cleburne* as it did. The hard question is this: Why did the Court ever burden itself with an unwieldy and mechanical three-tiered equal-protection scheme, which has no ascertainable roots in the equal-protection clause and no clear relation to the underlying principles served by the clause?

We think the answer lies primarily in the Supreme Court's desire to avoid adjudication that looks too "political." Strict scrutiny and intermediate review, the Court has suggested, are justified to protect classes of persons, such as racial minorities, that have historically been excluded from, or inadequately represented in, the political process (Ely 1981). Thus, when the political process has failed to represent the interests of a minority, the Court intervenes. On the other hand, when government disadvantages persons who have historically been able to look out for themselves through electoral politics, the Court typically assumes that a fair process must have produced a fair substantive result.

These theories seem to divide the judicial task of guarding the integrity of the political process from the political task of setting substantive policies. But as many commentators have shown, the supposed avoidance of substantive choices that such theories seem to offer is illusory (Cox 1981; Dworkin 1985, 57–71; Estreicher 1981; Tribe 1980). For example, persons addicted to intravenously administered drugs, lesbians and gay men, and aliens could all be considered under-represented in or excluded from the political process. The question of which, if any, of these groups merits special judicial protection cannot be decided without smuggling in substantive judgments about the characteristics and behavior of members of these groups.

Moreover, laws disadvantaging constitutionally protected classes are not *conclusively* invalid; at least in theory, the Court just closely examines them to see if they genuinely advance a legitimate and sufficiently important state interest. Is the suppression of homosexuality to promote a particular vision of public morality a state interest of this character? Is the criminal punishment of drug use driven by compulsive addiction such a state interest? These questions inevitably concern substantive problems of political philosophy.

That three-tiered review represents an attempt to distance judicial action from political considerations can also be seen in the Court's cumbersome efforts to avoid asking explicitly whether the good achieved by a governmental action justifies the harm inflicted on the disadvantaged class. The Court, apparently concerned that such balancing would look overly "subjective," and therefore insufficiently judicial, takes account of the harm inflicted by an action challenged under the equal-protection clause only in a clumsy and mechanical way. To be valid under strict scrutiny, for example, the Court must find that a racial classification is necessary to achieve a compelling state interest. Under the Court's structure, apparently *all* racial classifications are valid only if they accomplish the apparently fixed measure of good reflected in the word "compelling."

Logically, this approach makes sense only if all racial classifications offended equality in the same way and to the same extent. We believe that this is not so, that racial classifications employed in affirmative-action programs, for example, are legitimately measured by a moral calculus quite different from that properly applied to the prejudice-driven racial segregation at issue in *Brown* (Dworkin 1978, 223–39). The same problem arises for sex discrimination. Governmental classifications by sex are valid only if substantially related to an important objective: whether the classification is supported by biological differences between the sexes, by efforts to remedy the historical oppression of women, or by mere prejudice and stereotyping (Law 1984).

Justice Stevens's method, in contrast, asks the more sensible question of whether "the adverse impact" of government action "may reasonably be viewed as an acceptable cost of achieving a larger goal." That question need not lead the court into legislating; it demands only that governmental action be reasonably justifiable on grounds other than prejudice. For legislation that can be justified in this way, the further question of whether the legislation, in fact, advances appropriate goals at an acceptable cost is for political lawmakers.

Without the new directions charted by *Plyler* and *Cleburne*, the Court's standard equal-protection jurisprudence would be seriously inadequate for cases involving people with AIDS, or people who carry HIV. As a class, such people have many of the same characteristics as groups that the Court has formally recognized and protected through "strict scrutiny" or "intermediate review." Most persons carrying HIV, for example, belong to feared or disliked groups: gay men, or intravenous drug users and their sexual partners and children, who are disproportionately black or Hispanic. And members of these groups, once known to carry HIV, are obviously even more likely to suffer from irrational prejudice. Such persons are consequently in very real danger of having the executive and legislative branches act against them unfairly.

Nonetheless, the government undoubtedly could treat persons who carry HIV differently from others for some purposes. It plainly could, for example, prohibit a person who knows that he or she has HIV from donating blood. But because HIV is not spread through casual contact, in our view the government could not, for example, constitutionally refuse to employ HIV-positive persons. In short, some governmental classifications by HIV status are consistent with equal concern and respect for people with AIDS or HIV. Other such classifications, however, are not, and should be unconstitutional for that reason.

Given these facts, the Court's traditional structure leaves it poorly equipped to deal with constitutional cases involving people with AIDS or HIV-positive persons. Because HIV-positive status is relevant to some governmental actions, the Court would under its classical analysis almost certainly decline to apply strict scrutiny or intermediate review to classifications involving the status. Furthermore, the Court's typical reluctance to examine carefully the harm inflicted by a challenged action would seriously compromise its ability to decide cases involving HIV-positive persons in a realistic way. In short, if equal-protection cases involving discrimination against people with AIDS or HIV, when and if they arise, are simply stamped "rational-basis review" and given only peremptory consideration, then the prospects for real justice in this area are dim indeed.

Plyler and *Cleburne* offer a way out of the Court's usual understanding of the equal-protection clause. Those cases both involved classifications that are legitimately relevant to some governmental actions. Undocumented status, as we have said, is certainly relevant to immigration-related decisions, and mentally retarded status is relevant to a wide variety of state decisions involving education, benefit programs, and other matters. But in *Plyler* and *Cleburne*, the government applied these classifications unreasonably. The challenged governmental actions would not have discernibly reduced unlawful immigration or protected the well-being of the retarded, and would certainly have inflicted disproportionate harm on already disadvantaged people. Such harm could not, in Justice Stevens's formulation, be "reasonably viewed as an acceptable cost" in light of the insubstantial or nonexistent benefits of the challenged actions.

These two cases raise the encouraging possibility of a more coherent and less fragmented approach to questions of individual rights. Such a jurisprudence would not focus so insistently on the category of individuals that the government has disadvantaged. It would give greater weight to how the government has actually employed a particular classification. *Plyler*, it must be admitted, was a fragile five-to-four decision that the Supreme Court as now constituted might well decide differently. And in *Cleburne* the equities of the case were extraordinarily compelling; *Cleburne's* influence as a precedent in more difficult situations may be limited. Nonetheless, *Plyler* and *Cleburne* illustrate the way in which a more thoughtful and valuable doctrine of equal protection could be developed — to the benefit of, among others, people with AIDS and HIV infection.

Even if the Supreme Court were to develop and extend *Plyler* and *Cleburne*, the resulting doctrine would limit government conduct only, not the behavior of private persons. A multitude of state constitutional provisions and federal, state, and local regulations regulating public and private actions, however, also implicate principles of equality. The Supreme Court's constitutional decisions have plainly influenced many of those laws: *Brown*, for example, certainly affected the Civil Rights Act of 1964. The vision of equality that we believe *Plyler* and *Cleburne* support — whether or not it takes permanent root in federal constitutional law — is relevant for lawmakers considering antidiscrimination measures, for judges interpreting those measures, and for judges interpreting state constitutions. It is critical for the fair legal treatment of

HIV-positive persons—and many others—that the broad lessons of *Plyler* and *Cleburne* be fully absorbed and understood.

AIDS: The Forging of a Consensus

In the beginning—the summer of 1981—the phenomenon we now call AIDS had no name and no known cause, and appeared to affect very small numbers of people. Within a year it became clear that the disease was far more than a scientific curiosity; it was transmissible and spreading, and extraordinarily deadly. Associated at first almost exclusively with gay men, the disease acquired a name indicating that association—gay-related immune deficiency, or "GRID." As the caseload grew past 1,000, gay organizations and leaders in New York, San Francisco, and Los Angeles took note of this grim development, and began to contemplate and discuss the medical and political consequences of such an epidemic for gay people. A group of gay men in New York created an organization called Gay Men's Health Crisis to provide advice and services to those in need, and to engage in advocacy (Shilts 1987). The National Gay Task Force and other gay organizations established links to the scientists and officials studying the epidemic. Among other things, they helped convince the Centers for Disease Control that the term "GRID" was misleading and inappropriate, and the disease was renamed "AIDS," for acquired immunodeficiency syndrome.

Their effort to substitute "AIDS" for "GRID" was evidence of a larger concern: that the new illness would exacerbate the stigmatization already accorded gay people in the United States. Gay advocates also argued for more scientific and medical resources. Government, it must be recorded, was appallingly slow to respond (Shilts 1987). But both on principle and out of concern for the fight against the illness itself, they devoted considerable energy to the issue of the discrimination they believed AIDS would trigger.

In New York, these advocates looked in large measure to the state and city disability-discrimination laws.[25] In the fall of 1983—barely

---

[25]N.Y. Exec. Law §§ 292(21), 296 (McKinney 1982 and Supp. 1989); New York City Charter and Administrative Code: New York City Administrative Code §§ 8-108, 8-109 (Williams 1986).

two years after the disease was first identified — and in response to concerns about possible discrimination, the New York State Division of Human Rights issued a statement declaring that discrimination related to AIDS was prohibited by the state's disability statute (New York State Division of Human Rights 1983). The division asserted that the law covered not only people with full-blown AIDS, but also individuals "perceived" to have AIDS, those belonging to a group "perceived to be particularly susceptible to AIDS," and those related to or living with someone with AIDS. By the end of 1983, the division had received two formal complaints alleging discrimination on account of AIDS. The next year brought six complaints. By October of 1986, there were more than 30 reports or complaints (Eisnaugle 1986).

Shortly after the division's announcement, in October of 1983, Lambda Legal Defense and Education Fund, a gay-rights advocacy group, brought the first lawsuit alleging discrimination linked to AIDS.[26] The landlord who leased office space to Joseph A. Sonnabend, a physician practicing internal medicine in New York City's Greenwich Village, had tried to evict Dr. Sonnabend from his office because he treated patients with AIDS there. Lambda, in tandem with the state attorney general's office, argued on his behalf that those patients were "disabled" under the New York statute, and that the attempted eviction amounted to illegal discrimination against them. A New York City civil court judge issued a preliminary ruling in December in Dr. Sonnabend's favor, which constituted the first application by any judge in the country of a disability or handicap-discrimination statute to the new epidemic. (After the ruling, the parties settled the suit to Dr. Sonnabend's satisfaction.)

Two related scientific developments — the identification of HIV as the probable underlying cause of AIDS in the spring of 1984, and the approval by the Food and Drug Administration one year later of a test for the presence of antibodies to that virus — while encouraging from the perspective of medical research, significantly increased the potential for discrimination. Until the antibody test, people with AIDS were identifiable only through their history of symptoms associated with AIDS. In addition to simplifying efforts to diagnose AIDS, the test permitted identification of those who had been infected, but had no

---

[26]*People v. 49 West 12 Tenants Corp.*, Index no. 43604/83 (N.Y. Civ. Ct. N.Y. Co. 1987).

present symptoms of disease. In the hands of an employer, a landlord, or an insurance company with a discriminatory motive, a positive antibody test could result in serious harm to the person tested.

Gay advocates in California, fearing widespread discrimination as a result of the licensing of the test, went beyond reliance on the state's existing handicap-discrimination statute. They asked the state legislature for a specific statute to address the issue, arguing that without such protection, many gay men, among others presumed to be "at risk," would decide not to be tested. Their arguments succeeded. In the spring of 1985, the California legislature approved, and Governor Deukmejian signed, a bill outlawing HIV-antibody testing without the consent of the subject and specifically barring discrimination on account of HIV status by employers and insurance companies.[27]

In the fall of 1985, an increasingly aware public (affected in part by the disclosure that Rock Hudson was dying of AIDS) became witness to a sudden cascade of articles, programs, and conferences on AIDS. Many of these presentations speculated that the epidemic might spread significantly beyond the groups identified as at special risk. No longer did the disease seem confined to the remote worlds and "unspeakable" acts associated with gay men and drug users. The emergence of AIDS in young children—most of whom contracted the illness through blood transfusions or before birth from their mothers—made AIDS seem a more palpable threat to "ordinary" and "innocent" Americans. And medicine still offered little hope, except for the alleviation of pain. In these circumstances, how would the public and the politicians react?

In 1930, perhaps even in 1950, such a scenario would almost certainly have led to systematic coercion and discrimination: widespread loss of livelihood, forcible testing and treatment, mass detention, or worse. But in 1985 it did not. Some voices did call for compulsory measures. William F. Buckley, Jr. (1986), for instance, suggested that every person with a positive antibody test be marked on the buttocks with a distinctive tattoo. Followers of Lyndon Larouche gathered signatures in California for a "Prevent AIDS Now" ballot initiative, which appeared to authorize, among other things, a quarantine of HIV-positive persons (Kohorn 1987). (It failed at the polls in the fall of 1986.) By and large, however, politicians, judges, and administrators turned away from draconian proposals.

---

[27] 1985 Cal. Stat. ch. 22, § 1 (codified as amended at Cal. Health and Safety Code § 199.22a (West Supp. 1989)).

Two opinions rendered during this period are instructive. In December of 1985, the Florida Commission on Human Rights issued the first ruling in the country concerning the dismissal from employment of someone with AIDS.[28] The Broward County Office of Budget and Management Policy had fired Todd Shuttleworth, an intern with a satisfactory work record, because he had developed Kaposi's sarcoma, a skin condition associated with AIDS. Shuttleworth claimed he was able and willing to perform the duties of the job. The county based its dismissal on fear of transmission of the virus to others; it alleged that there was a general "lack of knowledge as to the severity and communicable aspect" of AIDS and that it could not risk even a slight possibility that another person would contract the virus. The commission totally rejected the county's arguments. Under Florida's handicap-discrimination statute, any risk of infection would have to be "substantial," the commission said, and the county had been unable to show even a "reasonable probability that AIDS can be transmitted by casual contact that commonly occurs in the workplace."

In New York City two months later, a state judge rendered his decision in a suit brought by parents seeking to keep children with AIDS out of the public schools.[29] The trial had taken five weeks. Eleven medical experts had testified. Because of the importance attached to the case by the city, the corporation counsel—the head of its law department—had personally conducted the defense. Like the Florida commission, the New York judge rejected fully the arguments in favor of discrimination. He ruled that under the federal disability statute—the Rehabilitation Act of 1973—the board was compelled to admit not only children with full-blown AIDS, but also children with asymptomatic HIV infections and children viewed as having AIDS or HIV infection, whether they actually did or not. He also held that the parents' request to exclude children with AIDS violated the equal-protection clause of the federal Constitution because it would be irrational to bar those children, but not children who were merely antibody-positive. (The parents had requested the exclusion of children only with fully developed AIDS.) The judge wrote:

---

[28] *Shuttleworth v. Broward County Office of Budget and Management Policy*, 2 Empl. Prac. Guide (CCH) ¶ 5014 (Fla. Comm. on Human Relations Dec. 1, 1985).
[29] *District 27 Community School Board v. Board of Education*, 130 Misc.2d 398, 502 N.Y.S.2d 325 (N.Y. Sup. Ct. 1986).

Although this Court certainly empathizes with the fears and concerns of parents for the health and welfare of their children within
the school setting, at the same time it is duty bound to objectively
evaluate the issue of automatic exclusion according to the evidence
and not be influenced by unsubstantiated fears of catastrophe.

These two opinions demonstrate how far the law had advanced in
the three decades before the onset of the virus. The two statutes relied
upon — Florida's handicap-discrimination statute and the federal Rehabilitation Act — did not exist before 1973. And the constitutional
analysis offered by the New York court would probably have been seen
as preposterous before the revolution in Supreme Court jurisprudence
since World War II.

Of course, both judicial decisions and legislative actions are merely a
part of the political culture from which they arise. In the AIDS epidemic, several factors promoted some degree of responsiveness to the
issue of discrimination. One was that the disease first arose among gay
men — a group traditionally viewed with distaste and scorn by most
Americans, but one also including many educated, affluent people
with some degree of political sophistication and personal influence.
More important, groups representing the afflicted had significant allies
in trying to persuade the government that oppressive measures against
HIV-positive people would only make the epidemic worse. By the fall
of 1985 the weight of public health opinion strongly favored voluntary
measures over coercive ones — even though there still remained some
scientific uncertainties about HIV transmission, such as the percentage
of people with HIV antibodies who would ultimately develop AIDS itself and the actual risk of infection through unintentional hypodermic
punctures. Witness this revealing passage from the first report in 1986
of the Committee on a National Strategy for AIDS of the National
Academy of Sciences' Institute of Medicine (1986), probably the most
prestigious panel to speak on the epidemic:

> The active voluntary cooperation of individuals who are at risk will
> be needed to curtail the epidemic. Coercive measures will not solicit
> this cooperation and could prevent it. Believing that coercive mea-
> sures would not be effective in altering the course of the epidemic,
> the committee recommends that public health authorities use the
> least restrictive measures commensurate with the goal of controlling
> the spread of infection.

The phrase "least restrictive measures" in this passage echoes well-known passages from civil liberties cases decided by the Supreme Court. That the Court's rhetoric should reappear here suggests the degree to which its efforts since 1950 to advance individual rights had become a part of our national conscience.

As already stated, this view of AIDS and public health is unquestionably tied to some degree to the vigorous advocacy of gay rights groups and their allies in the earliest years of the epidemic. But lobbying alone cannot account for the startling shift in attitude from previous epidemics. After all, gay rights groups were and still are small in membership and resources, and have been generally unable to achieve other goals on their agenda, except at the municipal level. And the shift by the public health experts has been too profound; in no previous epidemic had they expressed a collective preference for the "least restrictive" measures of controlling infection, and in no previous medical emergency had they put forward the view that the government should "solicit the cooperation" of those infected.

Such a dramatic change must have a more fundamental explanation. We believe that the legal and social revolution of the 1950s, 1960s, and 1970s created a climate in which the advocacy of gay rights groups and others could be effective – an atmosphere in which arguments made on behalf of the groups most affected would seem more than self-interested. The cases and statutes discussed in this article served, among other things, to direct the country's attention to the importance of fair treatment, encouraging educated Americans to think more deeply about the appropriate interplay between government and private institutional authority on the one hand and individual needs and interests on the other. When is discrimination justifiable? What does the state have to prove in order to engage in a discriminatory or coercive act? Must it try less drastic measures first? How does discrimination relate to public health concerns? The constitutional principles developed by the Supreme Court, as well as the discrimination statutes from the 1960s and 1970s, require that questions of this kind be explored in some depth. They force more careful and more rational thoughts. When the advocates asked these questions of scientists and public health officials in the first few years of the epidemic, they found an audience willing to consider them seriously.

By the time the public awoke to the scope and peril of the AIDS epidemic toward the end of 1985, a consensus against coercive measures and in favor of voluntary ones had already emerged among the experts (Gostin, Curran, and Clark 1987). They and the advocates for people with AIDS conveyed that consensus to the judges and administrators. And these judges and administrators, through opinions and actions like those described above, themselves reinforced the emerging consensus, helping to reassure and calm the general public. Only later did most legislative bodies begin to address AIDS, and by then the general approach had already been largely set.

The consensus eventually reached even the commission created by President Reagan in 1987 to advise the federal government on the epidemic. The president's announcement of his initial appointments to the commission was received with dismay by most experts and advocates for people with AIDS because the list included few who were knowledgeable about AIDS and also because it had a distinctly one-sided sociopolitical cast. The final report of a somewhat restructured commission, issued in the summer of 1988, contained, however, the following advice (Presidential Commission on the Human Immunodeficiency Virus Epidemic 1988):

> The primary focus in developing a comprehensive public health strategy to control HIV infection should be placed on those public health measures that are based on voluntary cooperation in risk-reducing behavior change.

The commission also spoke with conviction about the dangers of discrimination against people with AIDS or the virus:

> HIV-related discrimination is impairing this nation's ability to limit the spread of the epidemic. Crucial to this effort are epidemiological studies to track the epidemic as well as the education, testing, and counseling of those who have been exposed to the virus. Public health officials will not be able to gain the confidence and cooperation of infected individuals or those at high risk for infection if such individuals fear that they will be unable to retain their jobs and their housing, and that they will be unable to obtain the medical and support services they need because of the discrimination based on a positive HIV antibody test.

There is further evidence of the consensus against punitive or coercive measures. As of this writing, officials in 34 states have issued determinations, either administrative or judicial, that their disability or handicap-discrimination statutes cover AIDS, and in most instances HIV infection as well — an especially remarkable development in light of the fact that the first such declaration came as recently as 1983 (Gostin 1989; Leonard 1989). Legislatures in 29 states have enacted statutes to protect the confidentiality of HIV test results. Legislatures in 15 states have passed laws specifically outlawing discrimination on account of AIDS or HIV infection. And courts in several states in addition to New York have specifically upheld the right of children with AIDS to attend public school.[30]

What is even more significant, as of this writing no state has pursued any plan for mass detention or quarantine. Only one state has cut back a discrimination statute in response to AIDS. (In Tennessee, the legislature approved an amendment to its disability-discrimination law excluding "infectious or contagious" diseases generally [*AIDS Policy and Law* 1988].) And while discrimination unquestionably exists, systematic attempts to deny employment, housing, goods, or services to people with AIDS or HIV have been fewer than history would have led one to fear.

Exceptions and Deviations

That the most knowledgeable doctors, scientists, and public health officials have generally come to agree that compulsory measures would hinder rather than enhance the fight against AIDS does not mean that, over the course of the epidemic, the rights of the individual have invariably prevailed. In two areas in particular, civil rights or civil liberties questions have often been decided against the interests or desires of people with AIDS or HIV: government antibody screening, and the mandatory reporting of test results.

Government Antibody Screening

Most public health experts have opposed mandatory screening of the general public, or of segments of the general public (Gostin, Curran,

---

[30]*Ray v. School District*, 666 F. Supp. 1524 (M.D. Fla. 1987); *Thomas v. Atascadero Unified School District*, 662 F. Supp. 376 (C.D. Cal. 1987); *Board of Education v. Cooperman*, 105 N.J. 587, 523 A.2d 655 (1987).

and Clark 1987), and thus most legislatures have rejected such schemes. Two states, Louisiana and Illinois, dabbled briefly with compulsory testing for couples seeking marriage licenses, but in both instances the idea proved expensive and unproductive and was abandoned (Wilkerson 1989). Nonetheless, many states and the federal government have instituted compulsory screening programs for certain specially situated groups. The federal government has been especially aggressive on this front. It has, since 1987, methodically tested six categories of people subject directly to its supervision, with the general result that individuals with positive results are excluded: members and recruits of the armed services; applicants for immigration; volunteers for the Peace Corps; Foreign Service officers and their spouses and dependents; federal prisoners; and applications for residential placement in the Job Corps, a training program for poor teenagers (Gostin 1989).

At the state level, 14 states have engaged in the screening of prisoners, 6 among them segregating those with seropositive results. And 18 states have passed statutes permitting or requiring the testing without consent of any defendant convicted (or, in some states, merely accused) of a crime involving sex or drugs (Gostin 1989).

This testing without consent of certain special groups, both at the federal level and the state level, has encountered little opposition or complaint from either the public health experts or the public. Moreover, the few judicial challenges to their legality have for the most part failed.[31] Why has there been so little concern for compulsory testing of these particular categories of people, when the more general mandatory testing schemes have been seen as inappropriate? Lack of political advocacy may be one answer; unlike gay men, the groups tested are generally not organized in any political sense, and have few or no advocates to promote their perspectives. Moreover, all of the categories involve individuals who at some point engaged in an act setting them substantially apart from most other people; they applied for a special job—service in the Army or the Peace Corps—or requested an unusual benefit—residency in the United States as a foreigner or Job Corps

---

[31]*Local 1812, American Federation of Government Employees v. United States Department of State*, 662 F. Supp. 50 (D.D.C. 1987); *Batten v. Lehman*, no. CA 85-4108 (D.D.C. Jan. 18, 1986). But see *Glover v. Eastern Nebraska Community Office of Retardation*, 686 F. Supp. 243 (D. Neb. 1988), aff'd, 867 F.2d 461 (8th Cir.), cert. denied, 110 S. Ct. 321 (1989); *People v. Madison*, no. 88-123613 (Cir. Ct. Cook Co., Ill. Aug. 3, 1989).

training—or engaged in a crime. Some may believe that such individuals, by virtue of their special conduct, waive or forfeit any right to refuse or protest screening for HIV.

Such a belief does not, however, make the compulsory testing programs sensible, or even rational, as at least in theory they must be to comport with the basic constitutional principles developed by the Supreme Court. Screening Job Corps applications for HIV, for example, discourages participation from precisely the population of poor, inner-city teenagers the program was established to assist. Testing certain categories of federal workers goes against the central principle of handicap-discrimination statutes, especially the federal government's own Rehabilitation Act of 1973—that workers subject to disabilities should not be treated differently unless they pose a direct threat to others at the work site, or are unable to perform their jobs—and thus threatens to undermine that principle.

The way in which the legal concept of equal protection has developed since 1950 may help to explain the dichotomy over mandatory antibody testing: opposition to general screening proposals, but acquiescence to testing of certain discrete categories of people. The Supreme Court's jurisprudence of equal protection places great reliance on social classifications. Does the plaintiff belong to a "suspect" class? If so, some degree of "heightened scrutiny" may be appropriate; if not, the presumption is in favor of the government. Most antidiscrimination statutes rely similarly on special social or political categories. Perhaps the law's extraordinary emphasis in recent decades on categories of people in determining issues of individual rights has yielded the undesirable by-product of condemning those who fall into groups viewed with disfavor with significantly fewer rights than they really deserve—a sort of reverse strict-scrutiny test. Such disfavored persons—intravenous drug users, for example—should, we believe, be accorded an opportunity to have the rules that apply to them reviewed with full consideration of their rights and needs. As *Plyler* and *Cleburne* demonstrate, adjudication by category is often just too crude an instrument.

Privacy of Test Results

Certain privacy questions have also presented special difficulties in the history of AIDS to date. Four-fifths of the states, including all those most deeply affected by AIDS, permit people seeking antibody tests to obtain their results anonymously, generally at state-run clinics. Several recent studies indicate that some individuals will decline to be tested unless full anonymity can be assured (Fehrs et al. 1988; Johnson, Sy, and Jackson 1988). Eight states, however, not only do not make anonymous HIV tests available, but actually require doctors and clinics that administer the tests to report to state officials the names and addresses (and, in some states, the telephone numbers) of the people whose results are positive (Intergovernmental Health Policy Project 1989). The federal government has generally sidestepped the issue of whether such reporting requirements are appropriate; President Reagan's HIV commission endorsed compulsory reporting of antibody test results, but the Centers for Disease Control and the surgeon general have declined to take a formal position.

As described earlier, the Supreme Court's rulings on privacy have been rather opaque. While a federal constitutional right to privacy certainly exists, the Court has never formally defined — or offered a theory to explain — the right to privacy or personal autonomy. The Court's imprecision has made the resolution of issues like whether the federal Constitution permits states to require doctors to report names of patients who are HIV-positive very difficult, and has thus fostered division of opinion on these issues. In our view, the Court's failure to put forward a coherent conception of privacy has also given public health officials unduly broad latitude to collect sensitive medical information about individuals, permitting them to overlook or disregard studies showing that such schemes can discourage people from seeking care or treatment. In the absence of carefully developed constitutional principles surrounding informational privacy, the number of states compelling the reporting of personally sensitive HIV information is likely to grow.

Signposts to the Future

The response of most public health experts to AIDS, so at variance with the traditional approach to epidemics and other threats to the public well-being, underscores the profound changes in American legal doctrine and in American social attitudes wrought by the civil rights revolution of the midcentury, even though there are still shortcomings. Yet, the AIDS crisis has, we believe, done more than merely highlight previous developments. The crisis is of such significance, and the response to it of so extraordinary a character, that AIDS may itself play a role in the evolution of the concept of individual rights, both for lawyers and judges and for ordinary Americans with little formal understanding of the law. As in other ways, AIDS not only reveals changes, but may also promote them.

The AIDS crisis, as this country has confronted it, has the capacity to alter basic approaches to issues of individual rights in three ways. First, and most basically, this history of AIDS to date suggests that issues of discrimination, as well as questions about civil rights generally, are likely to be given very serious consideration in health crises to come — and perhaps in other kinds of crises as well. That is not to say that individuals will never again suffer unfair discrimination in the name of public health. But it does say that the issue of discrimination is not apt to be swept aside perfunctorily whenever an emergency arises, as has so often happened in the past.

Wars and panics as well as epidemics have all served at one time or another in the history of this country to justify significant incursions on the rights of individuals or groups. Traditionally, the mere invocation of an exigent circumstance has sufficed to explain the act of discrimination, with few voices raised in objection. After this country entered World War II, for example, President Roosevelt ordered the internment of more than 110,000 Americans of Japanese descent, supposedly because their national loyalty was in question (Mydans 1989). The detention provoked little public dissent or debate. And when the constitutionality of President Roosevelt's order came before the Supreme Court, the Court ruled that even under "the most rigid scrutiny," the internment was justified by the need to protect against the alleged threat of espionage during wartime.[32] The Court accepted at face value the government's assertion that the interned Japanese-Americans posed a threat to national security, without requiring that the government adduce credible evidence to support that claim.

The handling of the AIDS crisis points to the conclusion that such a similarly reflexive acceptance of discrimination is much less likely to occur, even during an emergency. AIDS is itself an emergency, threatening the health and well-being of millions of Americans across the country. Yet, public health experts have generally declined to propose

---

[32]*Korematsu v. United States*, 323 U.S. 214 (1944).

measures that would curtail the fundamental civil rights or liberties of those who carry HIV, even though such measures were routinely employed during epidemics in the nineteenth century and the early part of the twentieth century. The experts have largely accepted the arguments made by advocates for the people most affected by the epidemic that compulsory measures lead to needless deprivation and that such measures, far from advancing the public health, are actually apt to injure it. And, with the exceptions noted in the preceding section, government officials have acceded to the views of the experts. The present consensus may not hold together for the entire course of the epidemic, particularly as AIDS touches increasingly poor populations even further outside the American mainstream than gay men. But the consensus does still exist as of this writing and still does represent a new turn in this country's cultural perspective.

The second way in which AIDS may further transform ideas about discrimination emerges from the first. Before AIDS, many persons might well have guessed that during an epidemic of a transmissible disease, civil liberties and the public health were generally values in competition and tension with one another. Many people might also have thought that at a time of crisis, civil liberties would have to surrender to the public health—that the rights of the individual must succumb to the claims of the majority. The official response to AIDS has made plain that this simple opposition between civil liberties and public health is naive and misleading. As the passages quoted above from the Presidential Commission on the HIV Epidemic and from the National Academy of Sciences indicate, the public health experts have generally argued for a strengthening, not a diminishing, of individual rights, out of the view that the crisis will only worsen if the persons most in need turn away from the public health authorities and refuse to cooperate. As the President's commission urged, the "primary public health focus" has become "voluntary cooperation in risk-reducing behavior change," not forcible testing or quarantine.

Essentially, the experts have employed an ends-and-means analysis similar to those employed by the Supreme Court in its more thoughtful equal-protection cases applying "strict-scrutiny" or "intermediate" review. What is the end desired? What measures would help to achieve that end? If several means are possible, which one is the most narrowly tailored to accomplish the preferred result? The public health officials may not have known much about the Supreme Court cases, but they have nonetheless absorbed the general concern for the rights and needs of the individual that characterizes many of the Supreme Court's most important decisions since the midcentury.

The epidemic may have yet another enduring effect on the country's approach to issues of discrimination. In *Plyler* and *Cleburne*, the Supreme Court indicated a readiness, at least on the part of some justices, to reframe the constitutional doctrine of "equal protection of the laws" to reflect the actual diversity and complexity of bias. Those two cases demonstrate, for instance, that prejudice need not be rooted in centuries of class-based oppression to be invidious or material. The new conservative majority of the Court may choose not to develop further this strand of federal constitutional law, but, even so, *Plyler* and *Cleburne* may influence nonconstitutional cases and the interpretation of the state constitutions by state courts.

The AIDS epidemic has actually yielded very few constitutional decisions to date, since the disability-discrimination statutes—and cases like *Arline* that have interpreted those statutes broadly—have provided a simpler and less risky basis for litigants wishing to challenge discrimination against them. But AIDS nonetheless provides cogent evidence of the need to reconceive the constitutional doctrines arising from the fourteenth amendment along the lines of *Plyler* and *Cleburne*. An awareness of how discrimination hinders the struggle against AIDS—if government and courts are prepared to attend to that knowledge—may help bring the law to a yet more sophisticated understanding of the issue of state-based discrimination generally, and thereby serve the interests of the entire society.

References

AIDS Policy and Law. 1988. Tennessee Law Explained, Criticized at Bar Association. October 5.

Blendon, R.J., and Donelan, K. 1988. Discrimination against People with AIDS. *New England Journal of Medicine* 319:1022–26.

Brandt, A.M. 1985. *No Magic Bullet: A Social History of Venereal Disease*. New York: Oxford University Press.

Buckley, W.F., Jr. 1986. Crucial Steps in Combating the AIDS Epidemic: Identify All the Carriers. *New York Times*, March 18.

Caldwell, W.F. 1965. State Public Accommodations Laws, Fundamental Liberties and Enforcement Programs. *Washington Law Review* 40:841–72.

Cox, A. 1981. Book Review. *Harvard Law Review* 94:700–16.

Dworkin, R. 1978. *Taking Rights Seriously*. Cambridge: Harvard University Press.

————. 1985. *A Matter of Principle*. Cambridge: Harvard University Press.

Eisnaugle, C.J. 1986. New York State Division of Human Rights, AIDS Based Discrimination: A Summary of Reported Instances, September 1983–October 1986. New York. (Unpublished.)

Ely, J. 1981. *Democracy and Distrust*. Cambridge: Harvard University Press.

Estreicher, S. 1981. Platonic Guardians of Democracy: John Hart Ely's Role of the Supreme Court in the Constitution's Open Texture. *New York University Law Review* 56:547–82.

Fehrs, L.J., D. Fleming, L.R. Foster, R.O. McAlister, V. Fox, S. Modesitt, and R. Conrad. 1988. Trial of Anonymous versus Confidential Human Immunodeficiency Virus Testing. *Lancet* 2:379–81.

Georgetown Law Journal. 1973. Abroad in the Land: Legal Strategies to Effectuate the Rights of the Physically Disabled. 61:1501–23.

Gostin, L.O. 1989. Public Health Strategies for Confronting AIDS. *Journal of the American Medical Association* 261:1621–30.

Gostin, L.O., W.J. Curran, and M.E. Clark. 1987. The Case against Compulsory Casefinding in Controlling AIDS: Testing, Screening and Reporting. *American Journal of Law and Medicine* 12:7–53.

Institute of Medicine 1986. *Confronting AIDS*. Washington: National Academy Press.

Intergovernmental Health Policy Project 1989. HIV Reporting in the States. *State AIDS Reports* no. 7.

Iowa Law Review. 1965. Classification on the Basis of Sex and the 1964 Civil Rights Act. 50:790–91.

Johnson, W.D., F.S. Sy, and K. Jackson. 1988. The Impact of Mandatory Reporting of HIV Seropositive Persons in South Carolina. Paper presented at the Fourth International Conference on AIDS, Stockholm, June 12–16. (Unpublished.)

Kohorn, J. 1987. Petition for Extraordinary Relief If the Larouche Initiative Had Passed in California. *New York University Review of Law and Social Change* 15:477–512.

Koop, C.E. 1986. *Surgeon General's Report on Acquired Immune Deficiency Syndrome*. Washington.

Kurtz, P.M. 1977. The State Equal Rights Amendments and Their Impact on Domestic Relations Law. *Family Law Quarterly* 11:101–50.

Law, S.A. 1984. Rethinking Sex and the Constitution. *University of Pennsylvania Law Review* 132:955–1040.

Leonard, A.S. 1989. AIDS, Employment and Unemployment. *Ohio State Law Journal* 49:929–64.

Mydans, S. 1989. Aged War Detainees Still Unpaid for Lost Freedom. *New York Times*, Aug. 17.

New York State Division of Human Rights. 1983. Discrimination Based on

AIDS Is Prohibited by the State Human Rights Law. New York. (Unpublished.)

New York University Law Review. 1966. Age Discrimination in Employment: The Problem of the Older Worker. 41:383–424.

Parmet, W.E. 1986. AIDS and Quarantine: the Revival of an Archaic Doctrine. *Hofstra Law Review* 14:53–90.

Presidential Commission on the Human Immunodeficiency Virus Epidemic. 1988. *Report of the Presidential Commission on the Human Immunodeficiency Virus Epidemic.* Washington.

Risse, G.B. 1988. Epidemics and History: Ecological Perspectives and Social Burdens. In *AIDS: The Burdens of History*, ed. E. Fee and D.M. Fox, 33–66. Berkeley: The University of California Press.

Shilts, R. 1987. *And the Band Played On.* New York: St. Martin's Press.

Tribe, L.H. 1980. The Puzzling Persistence of Process-based Constitutional Theories. *Yale Law Journal* 89:1063–80.

Turner, R. 1988. Arline, Chalk, the Civil Rights Restoration Act, and the AIDS Handicap. *AIDS and Public Policy Journal* 3:23–28.

Wilkerson, I. 1989. Illinois Legislature Repeals Requirement for Prenuptial AIDS Test. *New York Times*, June 24.

Woll, J.A. 1964. Labor Looks at Equal Rights in Employment. *Federal Bar Journal* 24:93–101.

Notes on Contributors

Linda H. Aiken is Trustee Professor of Nursing and Sociology at the University of Pennsylvania, where she also serves as associate director of the Leonard Davis Institute of Health Economics. Health services and policy research, labor economics in health care, and medical sociology constitute her primary professional interests. Dr. Aiken is the author of the forthcoming volume *Nursing and Health Policy: Issues of the 1990s.*

Ronald Bayer is associate professor and A. Sheldon Andelson Am-FAR scholar in the Department of Sociomedical Sciences of the School of Public Health at Columbia University. He has written widely on the AIDS epidemic, the ethics of public health, and political controversies in health, science, and technology. Dr. Bayer is the author of *Private Acts, Social Consequences: AIDS and the Politics of Public Health.*

Charles L. Bosk is associate professor in the Department of Sociology at the University of Pennsylvania. In addition to the sociology of medicine, his professional concerns focus on the sociology of public problems and on law and society. He is the author of several works on the social management of medical practice and on physicians' attitudes in sociological perspective, including *Forgive and Remember.*

Nancy Neveloff Dubler is director of the division of law and ethics in the Department of Epidemiology and Social Medicine at Montefiore Medical Center/The Albert Einstein College of Medicine. An attorney, she specializes in gerontology and medical ethics in addition to health law. Ms. Dubler has recently published articles on improving the hospital discharge planning process and the moral dimensions of home care.

Harold Edgar is professor of law at Columbia University School of Law. The subjects of health law, law and science, and biotechnology figure prominently among his professional interests, along with the analysis of regulatory oversight of medical innovations. Professor Edgar is the author of a forthcoming article on AIDS legislation and medical privacy.

Renée C. Fox is Annenberg Professor of the Social Sciences at the University of Pennsylvania, with appointments in the Department of Sociology, the Departments of Medicine and Psychiatry, and the School of Nursing. A leading medical sociologist, her professional interests include the sociology of culture and science. Last year Dr. Fox published *The Sociology of Medicine: A Participant-Observer's View*.

Joel E. Frader is associate director of the Center for Medical Ethics at the University of Pittsburgh and teaches in the Department of Pediatrics at Children's Hospital of Pittsburgh. A physician, he works in the fields of medical sociology, pediatrics, and medical ethics. Dr. Frader is completing a study of the evolution of clinical medical ethics teaching and the ethical issues surrounding the critically ill newborn.

Richard Goldstein is arts editor of the *Village Voice*. He has written about popular culture, sexual politics, and the arts for the past two decades; in recent years, he has investigated and published numerous articles on the social, cultural, political, and medical aspects of the AIDS epidemic. His collection of essays on the 1960s, *Reporting the Counterculture*, appeared last year.

Suzanne C. Ouellette Kobasa is professor of psychology at the Graduate School and University Center of the City University of New York. A specialist in personality and social psychology, she works on issues of health psychology, adulthood, and individual difference. Dr. Ouellette Kobasa is currently directing a multi-year study of volunteers at the Gay Men's Health Crisis in New York City.

Carol Levine is executive director of the Citizens Commission on AIDS for New York City and Northern New Jersey. AIDS, biomedical ethics, and human subjects research are her major fields of professional interest. Ms. Levine is the editor of *Taking Sides: Clashing Views on Controversial Bioethical Issues* and the author of numerous articles on ethics and the AIDS epidemic.

Carla M. Messikomer is assistant professor of sociology in psychiatry at the School of Medicine, with secondary appointments at the School of Arts and Sciences, of the University of Pennsylvania. She works on the sociology of medicine, aging, and the relations between family, kinship, and ethnicity. Dr. Messikomer has coauthored an article on the role of family in geriatric rehabilitation.

Thomas H. Murray is director and professor at the Center for Biomedical Ethics of the School of Medicine, Case Western Reserve University. His professional interests focus on ethical issues in genetic engineering, the relationship among moral judgments, theories, and traditions, and the idea of community. Dr. Murray is coauthoring a report on ethics and genetic engineering for the British Medical Association.

Dorothy Nelkin is University Professor at New York University, serving in the Department of Sociology and as affiliated professor on the Faculty of Law. She has examined the interactions of science, technology, and society from numerous perspectives, in recent years focusing on the social construction of risk perception and on science communication. Professor Nelkin coauthored *Dangerous Diagnostics: The Social Power of Biological Information* with Laurence Tancredi.

Scott V. Parris is associate editor of *The Milbank Quarterly* and assistant secretary of the Milbank Memorial Fund. He has served as a consultant to the World Bank on sociological features of international development projects. Mr. Parris is the author of monographs on the evaluation of urban housing programs and social support networks among the urban poor.

Walter Rieman is engaged in the private practice of law in New York City.

David J. Rothman is Bernard Schoenberg Professor of Social Medicine and director of the Center for the Study of Society and Medicine at the College of Physicians and Surgeons of Columbia University. Among his current professional interests are analyses of innovations in medicine and their handling in regulatory processes. Dr. Rothman is the author of the forthcoming volume *Ruling Medicine: From Bedside Ethics to Bioethics*.

Victor W. Sidel is Distinguished University Professor of Social Medicine in the Department of Epidemiology and Social Medicine at Montefiore Medical Center/The Albert Einstein College of Medicine. He is a specialist in the study of equitable access to health care. The economic, social, and health costs of the arms race and the prevention of use of weapons of mass destruction are among Dr. Sidel's other professional concerns.

Thomas B. Stoddard is executive director of Lambda Legal Defense and Education Fund, Inc., and Adjunct Associate Professor of Law at New York University. An attorney, his professional concerns focus on civil liberties and civil rights and AIDS. Mr. Stoddard is the coauthor of *The Rights of Gay People*, an ACLU handbook now in its third edition, and has recently published an overview of the American response to AIDS.

David P. Willis is editor of *The Milbank Quarterly* and vice president of the Milbank Memorial Fund. A lecturer in the Department of Epidemiology at Yale Medical School, he has been active in the demographic, social, and epidemiologic aspects of health planning and policy. Mr. Willis coedited the volume *AIDS: The Public Context of an Epidemic* with Ronald Bayer and Daniel M. Fox.

Index

abortion, 194, 206, 210; and genetic counseling, 201–2, 204, 205; regulation of, 249
abortion rights, 191, 192, 199, 248
acquired immunodeficiency syndrome (AIDS): blood-related, 226–38; as disease of society, 1–14; efforts to control spread of, 194–5; as epidemic, 122, 242, 261–3; and individual rights, 267–9; response of law to, 244, 245–6, 248, 249, 250–63; social characteristics of patients with, 163–6, 167; symptoms of, 130–1; as total social phenomenon, 150, 161, 163–6
acquired immunodeficiency syndrome (AIDS) anxiety: representation in the arts, 39
ACT UP, *see* AIDS Coalition to Unleash Power (ACT UP)
adolescents, 7, 38
advocacy, 180, 181, 242, 256–7, 258, 261
affirmative action, 248, 253
age discrimination, 245, 253
AIDS: Cultural Analysis/Cultural Practices (Crimp), 18
AIDS and Its Metaphors (Sontag), 18
AIDS Coalition to Unleash Power (ACT UP), 36–7, 182–3, 184, 185; role of, 182, 185; tactics of, 182
AIDS Legal Guide, 58
Aiken, Linda H., 7, 9, 119–49
Alabama Federal District Court, 76
albumin, biosynthetic, 234
Alien (film), 23
Altman, Dennis, 175, 184
altruism, impersonal, 224
American Blood Supply, The (Drake, Finkelstein, Sapolsky), 223

American Cancer Society, 180
American College of Obstetrics and Gynecology, Committee on Obstetrics, Maternal and Fetal Medicine and Gynecologic Practice, 205
American Council of Education–University of California, Los Angeles Cooperative Institutional Research Program, 127–8
American Foundation for AIDS Research (AmFAR), 96
American Nurses' Association, 120, 137
American Red Cross, 180
Americans with Disabilities Act, 246
amniocentesis, 196, 209
And the Band Played On (Shilts), 24
Andre's Mother (play), 30
Andrews, Lori, 202
Ann D. v. Raymond D., 62
Anna Karenina (Tolstoy), 46
Annas, George, 210
antiabortion movement, 207, 210
antibody screening, government, 263–5
antibody test, 257–8
antidiscrimination measures, 245, 255–6, 258–60, 261, 265
Arkansas, 225
Arno, Peter, 175, 183
Arrow, Kenneth, 224
Arrowsmith (Lewis), 17
art, AIDS in, 8, 20–1
arts, response to AIDS in, 17–42
As Is (play), 18, 31
Asch, Adrienne, 200
Association for Drug Abuse Prevention and Treatment (ADAPT), 185
associations, American, 10
At Risk (Hoffman), 18, 28–9
Atwood, Margaret, 65
Audio 2, 25

277

M